ICD Connection:
Living with an implantable cardioverter defibrillator

A Collection of Patient & Family Stories

Helen McFarland, RN

Foreword by Frank Pelosi, Jr., MD

Cover Design by Donna Wilkin

Published by MPublishing, University of Michigan Library

Content available online at http://open.umich.edu/

ISBN-13: 978-1-60785-274-2

DEDICATION

This book is dedicated to all the patients and family members I have had the privilege and honor to care for during my years as a cardiology nurse. In some way, you have helped me to become a better nurse and a better person. Through you, I am continuously reminded to appreciate the strength and resiliency of the human spirit.

CONTENTS

FOREWORD

If you are reading this book, your life or the life of someone you know has likely changed or is about to change. The stories you will read are about change. These lives have changed with a heartbeat--something we take for granted every second of every day. These stories are about a group of courageous individuals who have received a remarkable technology called an implantable cardioverter defibrillator or ICD. These are stories of suffering, grace, renewal and wisdom.

What is an ICD? It is a device smaller than a deck of cards that is implanted under the skin to treat life-threatening heart rhythms that can lead to sudden cardiac arrest. As the name implies, sudden cardiac arrest results in a sudden halt of one's normal heartbeat that can lead to death in a matter of seconds. An ICD functions like a paramedic implanted in the body, monitoring every heartbeat and delivering treatments if a life-threatening heart rhythm is detected. One of those treatments is an internalized shock that, though it lasts fractions of a second, can be quite painful. The ICD has evolved from a technology requiring open-heart surgery to one that involves little more than a 2-inch incision and local anesthetic.

Having a serious heart condition that needs a permanently implanted artificial device that shocks you is a frightening prospect. The men and women in this book have received this sobering news at an unfairly young age. Most of them have received this news when they otherwise feel very normal--even vibrant. They must deal with life issues that most of us face only decades later; issues with a profound impact that extends to their parents, spouses, children, and friends.

As you read these stories, I would like you to reflect on a few themes. First, these individuals have endured a period of both physical and emotional suffering. Their mind is pummeled with questions that at first have no answers: What if I get a shock? What if the device does NOT work? What can I do? What can't I do? Am I broken? Who will love me like this? How long will I live? How will I die? The control and self-reliance that they once had now seem lost as they enter into a period of profound weakness, anxiety, and perhaps depression.

During this time of suffering and weakness, a remarkable process begins. The person avails themselves to the perfected grace of others. Almost miraculously, the person sees the uncloaked love and caring of family, friends, and even strangers. Gradually, but certainly, they find that an acquaintance who shares their plight becomes a dear friend, a boyfriend becomes a soul mate, and doctors and nurses become brothers in arms. They now cling to a faith that had once been only a companion. A touch of the hand, a caring smile, or a passing comment becomes a lifeline as these individuals rise from their seemingly drowning darkness.

From this grace, renewal begins. In these stories, a new person is reborn. For one young man, fear is replaced by fortitude to compete in collegiate athletics. For another, it is the resolve to find her dream job. For another woman, it is the discovery of someone who will truly love her for who she is, ICD and all.

The last few paragraphs of each of these stories describe the lessons these men and women have learned and advice they give to others. Wisdom is defined as understanding the deeper meaning of our world's realities. What remarkable wisdom they have gained from their experience! To paraphrase a popular song, they have become better friends and spouses; they love deeper and speak sweeter. They have learned lessons that all of us should heed: that each day of life is a precious gift; that true strength lies in a reliance beyond ourselves; and that our success will not be measured by titles or bank accounts, but by how we love, forgive, and care for one another.

I would like to thank these brave men and women for sharing their lives with us. They have transformed their personal tragedy into triumph simply by carrying on with their lives. They are living inspirations to their families, friends and the medical professionals that are charged with their care. I know that by reading this book, you will be changed. I know that I have.

Frank Pelosi, Jr., MD, FACC, FHRS
Director, Cardiac Electrophysiology Fellowship
University of Michigan Medical School

PREFACE

Each year at the University of Michigan "Young ICD Connection Conference," ICD recipients and family members courageously and generously stand in front of a crowded room and share their unique stories of living life with an ICD or supporting a loved one who has an ICD. The room is quiet as the attendees, ICD recipients themselves or family members, connect and identify with the range of emotions the speakers experience as they unveil their personal stories. Year after year, the feedback from the attendees can be summed up in a realization that they are not alone in their concerns, their worries, and their fears.

The inspiration for this book came from this particular session at our conference. Connecting with others who are experiencing similar situations can help us find encouragement and hope in our own situation. I would like to sincerely thank Kathryn, Colin and Ryan, Erika and Bryan, Phyllis, Terri, Brett, Renee, Lisa, Michelle and Alvaro who agreed to tell their very personal stories in this book. Each of them wanted to tell their story in the hope that it may help others who are finding ways to cope with similar life changing experiences.

As a nurse who has provided follow-up care to ICD recipients for a number of years, I was interested in publishing a book that provided an outlet for the voice of the ICD recipient and family members. There are numerous books and articles available from a medical standpoint about ICD implantation. However, no medical book could help me to understand the impact an ICD could have on someone's life. This I learned from listening to my patients. I'm hoping this book will be a resource for medical staff taking care of cardiac and device patients and allow them to gain insight into the patients' concerns by listening to the patients' voices in this book.

I would like to acknowledge and thank Jasna Markovac, PhD, Senior Advisor of Publishing and Related Business Development at the University of Michigan Medical School for her expertise and guidance with this project. Jasna listened and led the way to making my vision of this book a reality.

Lastly, I would like to thank the planning committee of the University of Michigan "Young ICD Connection Conference." The committee is made up of staff from the University of Michigan Congenital Heart Center and Cardiovascular Center. These committee members take great care each year to maintain a program that provides support and education for ICD recipients and their families and to do this in a festive manner.

Celeste Balas, RN	Dan Bochinski, RN
David Bradley, MD	Theresa Davidson, RN
Brynn Dechert-Crooks, NP	Macdonald Dick, MD
Susan Duart-Digon, LMSW	Carey Fette, RN
Eric Good, DO	Laurie Hill, RN
Laura Horwood, NP	Frank Pelosi, MD
Staci Kaczor, NP	Mary Kozonis, MSW
Martin LaPage, MD	Erika Laszlo
Shannon Laursen, NP	Corey Ryder, CVT
Gerald Serwer, MD	Barb Shaltis, LMSW
Roxanne Smith	Rachel Thompson, CCLS
Donna Wilkin	

Brian Boron – Medtronic, Inc.
David Thompson – Medtronic, Inc.

Helen McFarland, RN
University of Michigan Hospital
August, 2012

INTRODUCTION

The inspiration for the book, *ICD Connection: A Collection of Patient and Family Stories*, stemmed from our annual University of Michigan Young ICD patient and family support conference. This conference, "The Young ICD Connection Conference," is a multidisciplinary collaboration and is coordinated and hosted by the University of Michigan Cardiovascular Center and Congenital Heart Center cardiology staff. This conference was established in 1995 when we identified that young ICD recipients (children, teens, and young adults) have physical and psychosocial issues unique to their developmental age and differ significantly from our older adult patients. The indications for ICDs were expanding at this time and many young individuals felt isolated and alone. Survey results from our support conference reflect overwhelmingly positive feedback for the morning general session where a panel of patients and family members individually share their personal ICD stories. Patient and family stories highlight how the ICD implant affected their life, their challenges and struggles along the way, and share what was and wasn't helpful to their moving forward and adjusting to life with an ICD. The opportunity for these patients to share their experiences and interact with peers who have had similar experiences can facilitate personal growth and wellness on their life journey with an ICD.

Theresa Davidson, RN
Laura Horwood, NP
(founding members of the Young ICD Connection Conference)

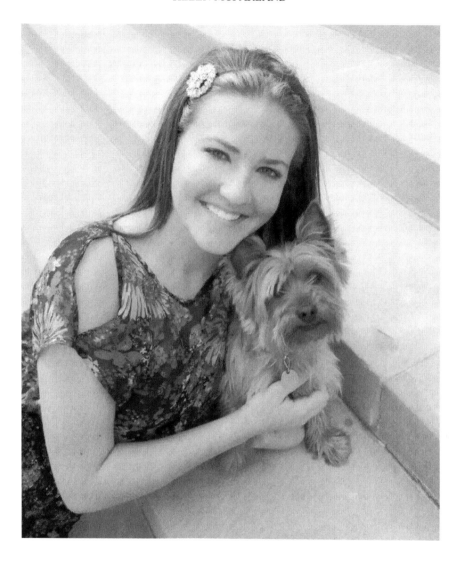

CHAPTER 1: A NEW WAY OF LIFE

Kathryn

If you saw me walking down the street, you would look at me and just think I was any other average teenage girl. I absolutely love to shop, I spend most evenings with my best friend Tyler, my cell phone is always within reach, I constantly check Facebook, and my Yorkshire Terrier Lincoln is my baby. If you stuck me in a group of people nothing would really make me stand out in the crowd, nothing noticeably obvious. One small scar though sets me apart from most people. That one small scar has impacted my life so much and is called an Implantable Cardioverter Defibrillator--such a big name for something that seems so small. It symbolizes what I've gone through and what is yet to come in life. According to Boston Scientific, an ICD or defibrillator, helps stop dangerously fast heart rhythms in the ventricles, the heart's lower chambers. To me, it's my life saver and I couldn't imagine life without it.

My life got flipped upside down over 10 years ago. It was my parents, my older brother, me, and my little sister. We were your average family living a happy life. The summer of 2001 though changed our lives forever. On May 28, 2001, my little sister, Alayna, suddenly and very unexpectedly passed away. The cause of her death was Myocarditis. It is a virus that attacks the heart. Alayna was only a month away from her 4th birthday when she died, I was 8 years old. She was my partner in crime and was my little shadow that followed me everywhere. We would rescue "wormies" in the rain, play in dress up clothes, or build these humongous forts with blankets and the

1

kitchen chairs. Alayna lived every day to the fullest and pointed out the small things that often times go unnoticed. She really taught my family to just slow down and enjoy life as it comes. Even though she is gone, she is never forgotten in our home. As quoted on her tombstone, "Those we hold in our arms for a little while, we hold in our hearts forever" which will always be held true with Little Miss Layna Ladybug. As much as no one wants to move on with life after a significant death, it seems that's the only way life can get any better. I was constantly scared the same thing was going to happen to me even though Myocarditis is neither contagious nor genetic. I remember my mom always reassuring me that nothing was going to happen to me. Much to everyone's surprise though that wouldn't be the case.

The summer after 5th grade was just like any other summer. I was enjoying school, Girl Scout camp, and hanging out with my friends. My mom decided to take me and my friend Kaitlyn out to get rewards from different arcades and food places for getting good grades on our report cards. We were having a good day and had decided to go to Chuck E. Cheese to get free tokens. I remember standing in front of this game, playing it and next thing you know I was waking up on the floor with my mom crying over me and paramedics surrounding me asking me questions like, "What's your name?" and "Do you know where you're at?" I was confused and scared out of my mind as to what just happened to me. I remember thinking on the ambulance ride, "I'm going to die, I'm going to die." All I could think of was what happened to my little sister, Alayna.

The only enjoyable thing about that ambulance ride was when the paramedic decided to play "paper, rock, scissors" with me. They decided at the hospital I had either locked my legs or had become dehydrated and I was released later that day. That week was stressful, but went by as usual and before long I was back to my normal self. Exactly one week from the day I passed out, it happened again while having a water balloon fight outside with my brother on the side of the house. I remember turning around to scream at my brother for hitting me with a balloon in the back and next thing you know I fell face first into the grass. I woke up to the world spinning and feeling my dad carrying me into the house. That night my parents decided it would be best to take me to Children's Mercy Hospital in Kansas City, Missouri. I was checked into a room that night, not exactly knowing what I was getting myself into. I was constantly monitored, poked, and prodded. I felt like 100 different doctors came into my room daily just to stick their cold stethoscopes on me and listen to my heart beat. It was rather annoying and at times I definitely was not happy. I have to admit, I didn't always have the nicest look on my face when doctors came in.

Every couple of hours I would get woken up as well so the nurses could check all my vital signs, not that I was getting that much sleep as it was. All these wires were attached to me to monitor my heart and if one came off, even just a little bit, the machine would start sending off this loud alarm. Also I had an IV going into my hand and I could only sleep a certain direction. I had to do a stress test much to my dismay. No one wants to have all these wires attached to them, and have to keep going faster and faster on this treadmill in fear of possibly passing out again. That was when my diagnosis was discovered, at the time I was diagnosed with Long QT Syndrome. According to the National Heart Institute, a problem with any part of the heart's electrical system can cause irregular heartbeats called arrhythmias. During an arrhythmia, the heart can beat too fast, too slow, or with an irregular rhythm. Faulty electrical signaling in the heart causes arrhythmias. My heart rate was getting up to a dangerously fast rhythm.

It was decided I would need to get an ICD and 2 days later, bright and early in the morning I was getting prepared for surgery. I was given relaxing medicine about 30 minutes before I was taken into surgery. My parents found that very amusing seeing as anything they told me I thought was hilarious, and I was practically falling out of my chair. In a joint effort, one had to prop my head up and the other had to keep me from sliding out of the chair. They were probably very relieved when a bed was finally brought in for me to lie on. On July 2, 2004 I had my first surgery. My last memory was lying in that bed, not being able to see straight. The next thing you know, I was opening my eyes to see both my parents standing there. I slept most of that day after I was out of surgery. The next day, in the afternoon I was released from the hospital, much to my excitement because it was the day before 4th of July and I just wanted to be at home with my family to watch the fireworks. My dad had to make a couple trips from the hospital back to the house because we had about 25 or so of those big balloons, tons of stuffed animals, and a couple vases of flowers. I remember sitting in the wheelchair with this huge bear in my lap spinning around in circles in the hallway waiting on my parents to hurry up. I was so ready to get out of there. That week was full of emotion and a whole new way of life for me. But I was ready to begin my 6th grade year.

Unfortunately that first semester in December, I had my first episode at home alone with my brother. I remember I started getting extremely nervous for no reason besides the fact my dad wasn't at home. I passed out for just a second on my bedroom floor and woke up to a shock, and my dog standing over me with a confused look on his face. I immediately got to my feet and ran into my parents' room where my brother was watching TV. I received 5 appropriate shocks in less than 5 minutes. After that scary event, I had difficulties returning back to school and pretty much stayed at home when I could. I managed to make it through my first year with the support of teachers, friends, and especially my family. It was like I was walking on a tight rope and I was losing my balance, but had managed to catch myself before I fell and I was able to keep moving.

Throughout the rest of middle school, I experienced 2 more episodes; each causing 5-6 shocks. Both of those episodes occurred during the 8th grade year. For those of you who have never received a shock, I can tell you what it's like. It is like someone punching you in the back extremely hard except it goes through your chest and you feel a tingle throughout your entire body. I have been conscious when I received my shocks, and I even have received a shock while hugging someone trying to calm myself down. Even though it's a scary experience that no one should have to go through, you'll be okay afterwards. I was shaken up but glad my ICD did what it was meant to do. Those shocks though emotionally hit me hard. That was where you could say, I completely fell off that tight rope. I couldn't go anywhere without my mom, every time I went on a walk I wanted to immediately turn around because I felt my heart rate was getting too fast. I had a huge fear of ambulances and I refused to stay at home alone. Even with my dad at home with me, I didn't ever want my mom to leave me or go anywhere. I would freak out when it was time for her to head off to work even though she would only be five minutes away. My anxiety pretty much took over and controlled my life. I really didn't know how life was going to go on. I never hung out with friends for fear of getting shocked again. All three times I received my shocks neither of my parents were around. I felt if I stayed at home or was always with my mom that nothing could ever happen to me. I buried myself into a hole, and I was scared to come out. Even though I had lost hope, deep, deep down I never lost determination and I think that is what kept me going. It got to the point where I just wanted to live life like any girl my age. High school was arriving and I wanted to make the best of those 4 years.

I really had a complete turn-around after a lot of hard work and struggle. I learned breathing techniques to relax myself if my anxiety ever started to go up. It helped tremendously. I still use that deep breathing today to calm myself at certain times and I definitely recommend others to use it as well. I was also put on anxiety medication which also helped a lot. But overall, I really had to change my mind frame and realize I couldn't allow my anxiety to live my life for me. It was choosing what I would do each day, and I couldn't let that happen anymore. Besides just coping with the anxiety, I also had to change my outlook on life. I was so angry that I was presented with this situation that a majority of people will never have to go through in their life. I was always looking at the negative side of things. I was upset that I could no longer go on those thrilling amusement park rides, I couldn't play any competitive sports, and I pretty much had absolutely no social life. I blamed my condition for everything and I felt it had completely ruined my life. I had to understand that you can't live in your life in anger. There was so much I could still do and half the things I couldn't do weren't because of my condition, it was because of my anxiety. Things I could still do definitely outweigh the things I could no longer do. Today, when other people start to become negative about something, I notice myself pointing out the positive side of things and I realize what an impact this whole situation has made on me and I'm happy.

I really couldn't have achieved anything without the support of friends and family, especially my parents who never gave up on me. My mom, who is my best friend, never once left my side and was always there for me even when she had to sleep in uncomfortable leather chairs night after night at the hospital and put up with my frustration of having to be stuck in that hospital bed. If you would have asked me five years ago how my life was, I would have said I hated my life and it was just so terrible. But I came to the realization; I was making this whole situation bigger than it needed to be. I am truly lucky. I have loving parents, a roof over my head, I'm well taken care of, and I can pretty much live a normal life, I was just allowing my anxiety to take that privilege away from me. If you asked me now how my life is, I can honestly say, I love it. Could I ever imagine being at this point in my life and be happy? No, but look where I am now. I graduated from high school last year with a 3.6 GPA. I have worked at the burger joint near where I live for close to 2 years. I attended the local community college this past fall. I have now decided to take a break from school and am moving to Raleigh, North Carolina to live with my great aunt. I am excited for this big change in my life and I would have never guessed in a million years this is what I would be doing today.

For those of you who haven't had an ICD very long or are struggling with accepting it, I can tell you things will get better. You may be sitting there thinking, "I don't believe what this girl is saying" because that is exactly what I would have been thinking 5 years ago. You just have to understand that this is an obstacle that life has presented to you. You can choose to go over or around it and continue moving forward or you can choose to stay stuck behind that obstacle and not get anywhere. Having an ICD is quite the learning experience. I had to accept that it is a part of me now and it's not going anywhere. I now enjoy showing it off to people and seeing their facial expressions when they feel my skin where that hard chunk of metal is inside me and I love telling people all about it. It is my life saver and I know that it will never give up on me, it's always going to make sure I continue living a healthy life. I should want to show it off and be happy for what I have. I received my second ICD over a year ago on a Tuesday. I was released the following morning and on Thursday I was back at school. On Friday night, I was back at work taking orders one handed. I didn't let my surgery slow me down or set me back at all. I have such strong determination after all that I've gone through.

This year will be coming up on 8 years since I first received my ICD. In total I have received 16 shocks, but the last shock was 5 years ago. This past year, my diagnosis was changed to CPVT after discovering the gene I had. It is a very similar condition to Long QT. It explained though why I had been shocked so many times because CPVT is a more aggressive condition. It is nice to know the gene I have, especially since I was the first person in my family to show signs of this heart condition. It was discovered that my mom also has the gene, but has not had any outstanding symptoms like me, and it was also discovered that my little sister had the gene as well. As of right now, my mom's side of the family is getting tested to make sure others don't have the gene. I am relieved to know that in the future when I have children, I will be able to know if they have the gene as well. I wouldn't change a thing about my life though because I believe that all I've experienced has made me a stronger, more grateful person. I have a more positive outlook on life now and look to the future with excitement, not fear.

To be completely honest, I'm happy life presented me with this situation because it made me realize you should always enjoy life. You never know when one day things may completely change for you. Life is hard. Every day can be a challenge. Getting up in the morning can be a challenge. Getting out of bed and putting that smile on your face during tough times is a huge challenge. But you need to remember, even through tough times, you can do it. There were so many times I wanted to give up, but I didn't and look at my life now.

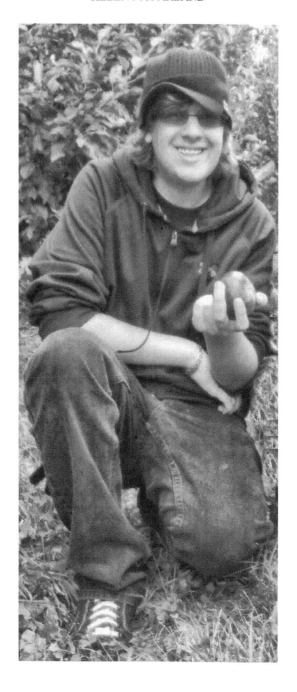

CHAPTER 2: CHEERING ON

Colin

My son Ryan was diagnosed with Ventricular Tachycardia in May of 2009. To date, the exact reason has not yet been identified. It has been over two and a half years and I am now just able to write about Ryan and share my story in hopes that it will help someone else find comfort. During those first years, I could not help but cry when I heard an ambulance siren or feel deep panic when my son's phone number showed up on my Caller ID.

Thursday, May 21, 2009, started out a normal day with our family of five: My wife Jennifer and our three boys Kevin then eighteen, Ryan thirteen, and TJ ten years old. That day would test our scheduling skills. Home from work and school with just enough time to eat and catch up with the day's events. Tonight we have to be in three different places with each of the boys. So the plan gets finalized. Jennifer would take Kevin to Career Night at the High School. I will drop off Ryan at Boy Scouts, and TJ will go with me to our Cub Scout meeting. It's a big event for the cub scouts as this is our season wrap up and "Cub-apolis," an Indianapolis 500- inspired race with seventy-five plus Scouts running laps in cardboard boxes all individually decorated. Weeks were spent planning, preparing and it was finally here. Will it go ok? Will the Scouts have fun? Are the parents going to behave? Sometimes competition brings out the best in some and the worst in others. As the evening unfolds, the excitement and fun is evident in all of the sweaty red faces. The Scouts are rewarded for their achievements and the leaders breathe a sigh of relief as the day comes to an end without incident.

My cell phone rings and it's my friend Tim on the other end, "Hey Colin, you better come over to the Church parking lot. Looks like Ryan collapsed from dehydration while playing "capture the flag." I responded, "Be right there Tim. TJ we need to go NOW." Hurrying to the Boy Scout meeting, I began thinking of past events where we have had to keep a close eye on the Scouts from becoming dehydrated. It can easily happen during a day filled with fun. We arrived within minutes and found Ryan laying in the parking lot and looking much worse than I had imagined. As I began talking to Ryan, my First Aid training started to kick in without even knowing it: Legs were numb, skin was cold and clammy, and his heart was pounding. He had thrown up all over. I shouted to Brian, "Call 911 we need help now." At this point, everyone realized this was more than dehydration and Ryan was getting worse. The EMTs and Police arrived in minutes. I was pulled away from Ryan to begin to recounting what had just happened. Quickly things progressed to what seemed to be a hundred questions. Does your son have a past history? Where has he been? Do you know if your son is taking drugs? This looks like he may have taken Ecstasy. You know, "E" is becoming a real problem with teens. I informed them that Ryan was not into that and we know his friends. That's not it. What is going on? Ryan was now on the stretcher and in the ambulance. The EMTs informed us that they were going to take him to Northwest Community Hospital and figure this out.

Fear began to take its hold. I frantically tried to reach my wife and son Kevin at the High School. Once, twice, three times. The calls went unanswered. Why won't they pick up? The school is notoriously known for being a cell phone dead zone. "Tim, can you take TJ home with you? I am going to the hospital and I can't get a hold of Jennifer or Kevin."

"You got it. No worries take care of Ryan." "Thanks."

Both the ambulance and I speed off. "Please pick up, please pick up." No answer. The sirens wail on ahead of me. "Is this really happening? What's going on?" The ambulance makes it to the hospital well before I do and now I struggle to find out where to go.

"Are you Dad?" "Yes, yes I am. That's my son."

They began cutting off his remaining clothes with a whole team scrambling around his bed hooking all sorts of instruments to his body. "Your son arrested in the ambulance ride over, but the EMTs were able revive him." Again, I have to describe what led up to this, past histories, drug use. "What's going on?" He's crashing again. It's like I am seeing a medical program on TV as I watch my son intubated, followed by CPR, and injections. "Everyone, CLEAR. Dad we need you now." The nurse grabs me by the arm, "Dad you stay here by his foot and keep talking to him. You don't let him go and we will do our part. Keep talking, he needs to hear you and let him know it's not time for him to leave." The doctors continue doing CPR, assisting his breathing, and increasing the levels of the defibrillator with each shock. He's flat lining and nothing is working. I was just cheering my youngest son to win a race, now I am cheering another son to live. "Ryan you need to fight. You can do it. I am here with you. Keep listening to me you can do it. Fight Ryan. Fight."

Twenty minutes pass and the nurse calls out, "I got a pulse. He's back with us. It's getting stronger. You did it Dad. He heard you. Great job." I am shaking uncontrollably at this point. Relief. Ryan is stabilized. I have to get a hold of Jennifer, still no answer. Finally, I get through.

"What? Where are you?" "At the hospital?" "Are you sure he's ok?" "Just get here quickly."

My wife arrived and again the story gets repeated. Now the doctor joins us and gives us even more details. We need to transport your son to Children's Memorial Hospital so they can figure out what caused this. It's decided that my wife will go in the ambulance with Ryan and I will follow.

Ok now where is the rest of the family. Hurried calls are placed to my Mom, Kevin, and Tim, "I need your help. We don't know what exactly is going on. We'll call you as soon as we find out something more."

Now almost midnight, I managed to call my best friend and tell him what has been going on. I totally break down and am sobbing in the car while driving. I have no idea how I made it to Children's Memorial hospital without getting into a car accident. Arriving at the hospital, I head to the ICU where the doctors began trying to figure what caused Ryan to go into cardiac arrest. At two thirty in the morning, Dr. Raj sat on the floor at our feet as we listened to him explain what had happened and what they are going to do," Looks like Ryan is stable, but we are going to keep a close eye on him." How unbelievably compassionate Doctor Raj is, looking up at us assuring they will do everything they can. My wife and I hold each other and look at our son. Was this really happening?

In the days that followed, test after test were performed; each one coming back negative. Great news, but what caused all of this? After nearly a week in the ICU, it is determined that because Ryan had a recorded EKG showing his heart beating at over 300 times a minute, the best course of action is to have an Implantable Cardioverter Defibrillator (ICD) surgically connected to his heart and start a course of medicine to allow him to heal and lower his heart rate. Ten days later and Ryan is finally released from the hospital with medicine, rules, and follow up visits scheduled. More information and events have transpired than we could possibly absorb.

So much information is readily available on the internet. Finding out as much as possible about the functions of the heart, causes of arrhythmias, potential reasons, brings a level of comfort and control. Seeing Ryan alive, smiling, and looking perfectly fine except for the four inch long scar on his chest quickly snaps me out of dwelling on all that has happened. It becomes clear early on that there will be no way I can be with Ryan at all times, so we make sure he is able to answer any question about his condition.

In November 2009, Ryan was at Boy Scouts when I received another call. "Colin, the ambulance is on the way. Ryan is awake and talking but his ICD went off." We follow the protocol taught to us and call the cardiologist and then go to the hospital. One of the EMTs recognized Ryan from May and they are able to catch up on what has happened since then. Ryan is in control with the help of his ICD. It is confirmed as an appropriate shock. We are released from the hospital after checking that the lead wires are OK and the device is working fine. We decided to have genetic testing done with hopes that it would reveal why. No luck. Negative.

Ryan continues to amaze us with how strong he is physically and mentally. Ryan is not the typical baseball playing type of boy. His interests were always more artistic in nature and he started playing the alto saxophone in junior high. Marching Band in High School is his love. In July 2010, during summer training for Marching Band, his ICD went off. Again, we are back in the ICU to see what is going on and why Ryan keeps having arrhythmias. More tests. All negative, Ryan's medicine is switched up to include a calcium blocker along with the beta blocker. With this new combination and the ICD, it is our best bet.

Ryan has been seeing a therapist since March of 2011 and we are continuing to heal, grateful each day to have all of our children with all of life's ups and downs. In October 2011, we were able to go to a conference in Ann Arbor, Michigan, the Young ICD Connection, and take another step forward. Next year, Ryan hopes to tell his story and meet more people like him. In the beginning, we were not sure that Ryan would have any kind of a future.

Today, our doctors seem like family and check-ups are more like reunions. As a parent, I will always have concerns, but now they are pushed to the back of my mind by hopes and dreams: Watching our son grow, learn to drive, graduate, go off to college, and beyond. I am so grateful for all those around us and those who we have met throughout the years.

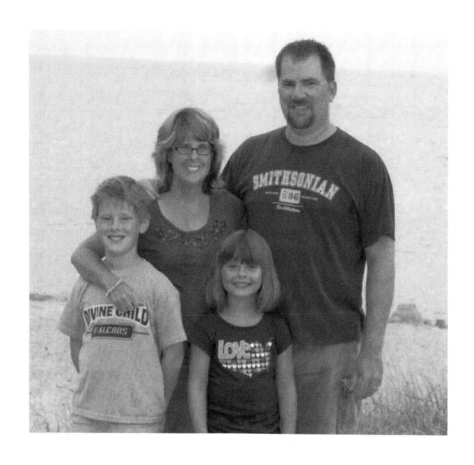

CHAPTER 3: IT'S A LOVE HATE RELATIONSHIP

Erika

I was born with a congenital heart defect called Tetralogy of Fallot. I had bypass surgery when I was two years old and open heart surgery to correct the defect when I was five. I was one of the first babies to survive both surgeries at the medical facility where I was being treated. Because of this, the physicians at the time did not know what my future would hold. They couldn't promise I'd see the age of ten, let alone have a family one day.

After my initial surgeries, I followed up with my cardiologist annually and had no restrictions on my activities. I played some sports and was very involved in extra-curricular activities at school. I never really thought about my heart condition. I did my best to make sure it wasn't an issue, but sometimes there were reminders. I'll never forget my sophomore year biology class. For some reason we were talking about open heart surgery and I mentioned that I had one when I was five. The teacher looked at me strangely and barely acknowledged my statement. Later that day at home, my teacher called our house. He let my mother know what I said. He honestly thought I made it up. I remember my mother spending some time explaining my diagnosis and what had happened to me when I was younger. The next day when I went to school, the teacher took me aside and apologized. He felt guilty that he thought I would make up such a story. He said that just looking at me, he would have never guessed what I had gone through as a child. I told him it's not something I talk about and I want to do my best to be as "normal" as I can. I appreciated the fact that he didn't make a big deal out of it and he respected my privacy afterwards.

When I was about twenty years old, my life changed drastically. I worked at a local TV studio and was getting ready for a live production when I suddenly became very lightheaded and dizzy. My heart was beating so fast it felt like it was going to literally pop right out of my chest. I was doing everything in my power not to pass out; I am not one who likes to cause a scene. Once the sensation went away I called my parents and told them what happened. They suggested I go to the ER. At the ER, they did an EKG and lab work and could not find anything wrong. Looking back on my experience, I wonder if the ER staff thought I was crazy or looking for attention. I was so adamant that they were wrong and they just shrugged their shoulders and said, sorry we can't find anything.

A few weeks later I followed up with my cardiologist. When I told her what had happened, she said it was possibly an anxiety attack or maybe it was all in my head. I was so offended by what she said. Anxiety attack?! In my head?! Are you kidding?! In that moment of frustration, I looked at her and said I was done. I asked her to refer me to another physician. I knew what happened that night was real and I needed answers. I needed someone to believe me.

Thankfully she referred me to an electrophysiologist, a cardiologist who specializes in arrhythmias. After meeting with him, he suggested I should have an electrophysiology study to find out whether I had an arrhythmia. The symptoms I described were similar to one, but he wasn't sure what kind. The day of the study I was very nervous since I didn't know what to expect. Aside from my yearly follow-up with the cardiologist, I had not had any major testing previously.

A few minutes into the study, they were able to induce an arrhythmia. I was feeling dizzy, lightheaded and my heart was pounding like it was going to pop out of my chest. I recall the doctor asking me if these symptoms were similar to the ones I had that day in the studio. I told him yes. I recall him being very calm and stroking my hair and telling me I was going to take a little nap and that we would talk again very shortly. Then everything went dark. Later, when I woke up I could hear my doctor talking to my parents. I heard words like dead, lucky lady and the statement, she really shouldn't be here. She should be dead.

That day we learned that I have ventricular tachycardia, a.k.a. sudden death syndrome. My heart was beating over 300 beats per minute in the lab and they had to defibrillate me three times to return it to normal sinus rhythm. Once the doctor realized I was awake, he came over and told me how lucky I was and the fact that I survived the first episode without any medical intervention was nothing short of a miracle.

I stayed in the hospital for about 4 weeks. They tried every drug possible to try to suppress the arrhythmia. I was in and out of the EP lab so often I lost count. At one point a cardiac surgeon came in to my room with a flip chart with fancy pictures and introduced me to the implantable cardioverter defibrillator (ICD). When he explained what an ICD was and what it would do, I told him pack up his stuff and get the heck out of my room. There was no way that device was going inside of me! I was stunned they would even think that was an option. I was still hoping there was a drug out there that would help me.

At one point my doctor was out of options and suggested I meet with a colleague in Philadelphia. I was transferred by air ambulance and once there I had yet another EP study. They were unable to induce the arrhythmia, which you would think was good news. The bad news is the drug that finally worked is not the kind of drug a young person should be on for the rest of their life. The side effects are brutal, such as organ failure and blue skin discoloration which is irreversible.

Once I came home from Philadelphia I met with my cardiologist again. He gave me yet another option. He spoke to two different physicians groups, one in London, Ontario and another in Texas. Both groups felt confident they could help me and were very eager to take me on as their patient. I chose London, Ontario because it was closer to home. My mother was coming with me and I wanted my dad to be able to travel back and forth on the weekends to visit. With all the issues I was having, they were still busy at home raising my brothers and sisters. We needed to be close by.

Once we arrived in London, I was greeted by some of the best doctors in the field of electrophysiology. I loved the fact they had a plan and that the guessing game was over. The plan was to do an ablation. They would induce the arrhythmia and try to ablate the scar tissue. It was determined that the arrhythmias were a result of scar tissue build up from the surgery that I had had when I was five years old. They explained to us that the ablation procedure had been successful in many patients and there was a good chance it might work for me. We were thrilled.

They did four ablations and none of them were deemed successful. They wanted to make one more attempt, but with the understanding that this time if they didn't feel confident the ablation was 100% successful they would implant an ICD. I remember saying, "an ICD"? What is that? Then I remembered the doctor who came to visit me with his fancy flip chart. I panicked. I thought this could not be my only option. All the research out there and my only option was a box with a bunch of wires that would zap my heart. No way! There is no way that is going inside of me. I cried and screamed until I was exhausted.

As a joke (partially) I asked my mother if Dr. Kevorkian would come to Canada with one of his contraptions. In that moment, I wanted to die. I can honestly tell you today that I wanted to die more than anything. I was done being pricked and prodded. I just wanted to escape my new found reality.

As I reflect back, I feel so guilty about my behavior toward my mother that day. She had been at my side the entire time supporting me emotionally and suddenly she became a verbal punching bag for me. I know it wasn't fair. I wish my dad was there to hold her hand and let her know that everything would be OK. Instead, she did her best to be strong. I know she broke down when she left my room that night. I can't imagine her alone and crying. I am sure she felt helpless as well. My mother has always been a positive person no matter what comes our way. She would always tell me that God never gives people things they can't handle. At first, I resented that statement. I wondered why God would do this to me. What had I ever done to him? I don't think anyone deserves what I have gone through in the last few months. I wouldn't wish it on anyone.

After my temper tantrum, the doctors sat down and explained I did not have a choice. If the last ablation did not work they would have to implant the ICD. They would not let me go home without it. What was I to do? I wasn't going to live in a hospital for the rest of my life and besides my insurance probably would not allow it either.

The next day I had my final ablation and this time they did it as an open heart procedure. When I woke up from the procedure, I remember reaching down to the left side of my abdomen praying that nothing would be there. I was disappointed to feel the tape and the packing that covered my incision. I knew that the ICD was implanted. I remember falling back asleep and tears falling down my face. I just wanted everything to go away. When I finally awoke it was explained to me that they ablated 99% of the scar tissue but 99% was not good enough for them. They felt they had no choice but to implant the device. For some reason, I felt someone owed me an apology for what they just did to my life. I sat there waiting for someone to say it but they never did. We just sat and looked at each other. It was a very awkward moment. At one point they went as far as to tell me that I probably would never need it. It was more of a back-up than anything else. That statement gave me hope. I desperately clung to their words.

I know doctors cannot predict the future but they were wrong. In the twenty plus years that I have had an ICD, it has saved my life nine times. Nine times! Can you believe it? It hurts like hell, but it has given me a gift, the gift of life. There aren't enough words in the dictionary to express my gratitude. Never in a million years did I ever think I would say that.

The first time the ICD fired it was horrible. I became paralyzed with fear and would not walk out to the car so my parents could take me to the ER. I felt that if I walked it would raise my heart rate and it would start firing again. I have never felt such fear like I did that day. After the initial shock, I barely left my house for three months. I was always afraid it was going to fire. I would sit in a chair and count my pulse all day long. I wanted to be ready if it was going to happen again. I did not want to be caught off guard. When I did leave the house, I always had to have a plan. If I was in restaurant, I had to sit by the door. If the ICD was going to fire, I needed to get out, and get out fast. One time my friends talked me into going to a movie and instead of sitting and enjoying the movie, I sat in the bathroom worried that my heart would do something funny and the ICD would fire. My parents would take me for car rides and I would lie in the back seat and just take naps. I would think, if I am sleeping, it won't fire. My heart is at rest so it won't beat fast enough for anything to happen. Once I attempted to venture out to a video store by myself and had an anxiety attack. My dad had to come and pick me up. I was admitted to the hospital so many times for anxiety, it's almost embarrassing. At one point, it was suggested I meet with a therapist. I was willing to give it a try. I was exhausted both mentally and physically, and I was finally admitting I needed help.

My therapist was the best. In the beginning, I would meet with her twice a week. She was very tolerant of my behavior and was a very good listener. She would give me small goals to reach each week. I remember one goal was to simply go to the movies and try to stay in my seat as long as I could. She taught me breathing techniques that I could use any time I felt anxious. She was wonderful. At one point she suggested I attend a support group meeting. I laughed and said, "No way am I going to sit around with a bunch of people that could be my grandparents. What could we possibly have in common?" After weeks of her asking me to attend a meeting, I did. I did it for my therapist, not necessarily for myself. I really needed her off my back.

When I arrived, I noticed I was the youngest person in the room and wasn't a bit surprised. Everyone was so kind and they were doing their best to engage me in conversation, but I just couldn't do it. I wasn't ready. I felt like I had this wall around me and I needed to protect myself. As I sat and listened to everyone speak that day, I was in awe over how much we all had in common. It really didn't matter how old we were. We all suffered from some type of anxiety due to the ICD. The difference between me and the group is that yes, they had anxiety, but they learned to cope. They learned that life must still go on. This meeting really changed my perspective. I remember the ride home that evening. I cried all the way home. I wasn't crying because I was sad. I was crying because I didn't feel alone. I had people that I could relate to and it gave me hope. I started to see the light at the end of the tunnel. I just needed a little more time.

I continued to attend the meetings and eventually I shared. I was no longer the scared girl in the corner who wouldn't speak. It was a great outlet for me and I learned so much about myself. It was so nice to express my fears and have others understand. As I sat and listened to others, I realized how much energy I wasted worrying about something that more than likely wasn't going to happen. It also made me realize how much I missed out on, and how unhealthy it was for me to continue living like that. I was mentally and physically exhausted. It was time for me to move on. I knew it wasn't going to happen overnight and I had to be patient, but I needed it to happen. I needed to enjoy life and be thankful.

I have had my ICD replaced numerous times over the years. The first time it was replaced I ended up with an infection. A few weeks after I was discharged, I spiked a fever and noticed a blister on my incision site. I went back to my cardiologist's office to discuss my symptoms and find out what to do next. My cardiologist was on vacation so one of his colleagues was following my care. Without doing any tests the doctor decided it was a "female issue" and that I should just go home. He blatantly ignored my symptoms and wanted to send me on my way. When I called my mom to give her an update she was appalled. She called another colleague in the office and begged for them to do an ultrasound. He agreed it was appropriate and would do it the next day. The ultrasound was done and they found the pocket where the ICD sits was infected. The infection was so severe that I was sent back to London, Ontario that afternoon. They said later that if I had waited another day or two the infection would of spread to my blood stream and I could have died.

They removed the ICD and I was put on I.V. antibiotics for four weeks. Since I was no longer protected against ventricular tachycardia, the doctors didn't want to risk it and they admitted me for the duration of the treatment. At this point, I was depressed. It seemed like every time I went two steps forward I went back four. Nothing was really going my way.

After I was discharged, everything seemed to be going well. Then one day the blister reappeared. Without even talking to the doctor I knew the infection had returned. I was so tired of the ICD and the problems it was causing that I just wanted it out. When I met with the cardiologist it was determined that the electrical leads that connect the ICD to my heart were infected too. I refused to go back to London and demanded that something be done locally. The doctors agreed to treat me and remove my ICD. I was tired of dealing with the issues and really needed a reprieve. The doctors removed the leads and the ICD with the understanding it would be for a short period of time. When it was time to put the ICD back, I refused. Emotionally, I wasn't ready. I wanted things done on my own time.

As time went on I started to date again. My relationships never really lasted because who wants to date a girl with a heart issue who has both emotional and physical scars? Then one day, I finally met the man I was destined to marry, Bryan. I wouldn't say it was love at first sight. At the time I was still leery about relationships and didn't want to commit to someone knowing it may not last. The first time we met I told him I had Tetralogy of Fallot and that I also had sudden death syndrome. I explained that I'd need an ICD implanted eventually and how much of an emotional mess it has made me over the years. I also told him about my scars and that they were not a pretty sight. To me it was like a little test. If he really likes me, he won't care and he will ask me out. If he doesn't ask me out, then it wasn't meant to be and I nipped that in the bud. Well, he asked me out and almost 3 years later we married.

Prior to that, though, about six months after the ICD had been removed, and not long into my relationship with Bryan, I was driving in my car on my way to play softball when I became lightheaded. I was dizzy and my heart was beating rapidly. I was so scared; I thought I was going to die. I didn't have my ICD which meant I didn't have a back-up. It took that one moment for me to decide I needed my ICD. I called my doctor and set up a surgery date for the next week.

I learned that Bryan was the one when my mother tried to give him an out during the ICD placement. Part of the workup to getting the new ICD included another visit to the EP lab for more tests. Bryan came along with my mother so she wouldn't have to sit alone. They wanted to put in an arterial line for the study. I refused to have the line inserted. Arterial lines are very painful and in the past they always inserted them after they gave me the anesthesia. This time they refused to do it that way. They finally gave in and gave me two different medications: one to calm my nerves and one to make me forget about the procedure, yet I was still awake. I don't remember anything, but I understand I was not a very good patient. Let's put it this way, my mother didn't know I could swear like a sailor. At this point my mom looked at Bryan and said, "We understand if you want to walk away. We know this may be tough to handle." Bryan's response was, "You can't help who you fall in love with and I am here for the long haul." My mother loves to tell that story, and she knew at that moment that he was the one for me.

Before Bryan and I married we agreed to meet with a high-risk OBGYN to talk about the possibility of having children. I was always told that I probably should not have children. It would put too much stress on my heart, and there was a really good chance that my children would be born with the same heart defect as well. After meeting with my OBGYN and consulting with my cardiologist, they both agreed it would be safe to try. About a year and a half into our marriage, our son Ethan Matthew was born. It was a tough pregnancy due to a partial placenta abruption which put me on bed rest for almost five months, but everything worked out well. Ethan was born almost 6 weeks early and weighed 4 pounds 4ounces. He was a very healthy boy. Four years later, almost to the day, our daughter Sophie Catherine was born.

My pregnancy that time was much different. I was able to work until the day she was born. Five weeks before Sophie was due I noticed a tremendous weight gain in a short period of time and called my doctor. As soon as I made that call, I knew that day would be her birthday. When I arrived at the hospital it was determined that I was in early stages of congestive heart failure. Almost 5 hours after I made the call to the office, Sophie was born via a C-section. She too was a healthy baby weighing in at 5 pounds 4 ounces. I was very fortunate because the congestive heart failure resolved itself on its own.

Since my marriage and the birth of my children, my anxiety is almost nonexistent. I still have my moments but they are not as often or as bad as they were years ago. I have learned to live and, most importantly, love and enjoy my life. I have a great marriage, career and am very involved with my kids' activities. When I share my cardiac story with others, they can't believe everything I have gone through. I look like a normal wife and mom with a full-time job who is doing her best to raise her kids and take care of the family. I love to hear that, because normalcy is what I strive for. I just want be normal. I know that without this ICD, I would have never had the opportunity to live this wonderful life I lead. I am grateful for my mother and father who never let me give up. I am thankful for my brothers and sisters, who I am sure felt neglected at times, yet they were so patient and loving. I am thankful for my wonderful extended family and friends. I don't know where I would be today without them. Last but not least, I am thankful for Bryan for loving me. We have been through some rough times but he has never wavered. He is always by my side and that is what makes it easy for me to get through the tough times.

Over the years I have been diagnosed with atrial tachycardia, atrial fibrillation, pulmonary hypertension and congestive heart failure. I have had my ICD replaced numerous times and battled a few more surgical infections. I had my pulmonary valve replaced a year and half after my son was born. Then a few years later diagnosed with endocarditis.

To the average person this may seem like a lot for one person to handle. But when I look back at my experiences, I think about the statement my mother would repeat over and over – God gives us what we can handle. As much as I resented that statement, I have grown to appreciate it. What God gives us does make us stronger. Because of this strength, I consider myself a survivor and will always be ready for what he will give me next.

CHAPTER 4: ME, MY WIFE, AND HER ICD

Bryan

My wife Erika has asked me upon occasion throughout the years if I regret anything about our life together. Asked in jest it still provokes reflection and calls for an answer. Marrying her wasn't as much a choice as it was finally finding my other half and grabbing on. Trite as it sounds, I can't imagine my life without her in it- nor do I want to. She was the only person that could have given me the family and memories I have now.

I think it helped that she started off being very frank about her heart condition. We weren't long into our first conversation when she brought up rather sobering concepts including sudden-death syndrome, Tetralogy of Fallot, open-heart surgery, ventricular tachycardia, arrhythmia, life-threatening infections and six-week hospital stays. She told me about the trials her parents and siblings went through as she endured myriad medical tests and treatments including repairs, ablations and placement of an implantable cardioverter defibrillator (ICD), disrupting their lives for weeks or months.

She told me how, after getting shocked by the I.C.D. for the first time, she never wanted to leave the house. When she did go out, anxiety would overpower her reason and she'd constantly worry, "What if it goes off, what if. What if" to the point of obsession, always having an exit plan. Once she went to the movies and worried so much that she went and hid in the restroom for the rest of the time. Erika underwent rounds of therapy in trying to cope with her new reality, developing the tools to live life despite the anxiety and depression.

When asked to describe what would have been the perfect woman for me at the time of our introduction, none of this would have been on my list, I assure you. How often do you hear the phrase "sudden-death syndrome" when you first meet someone and wind up getting married and starting a family?

Though she was between ICDs when we met, it wasn't long before I had my first exposure to Erika, the patient. I didn't know what to do but just be there despite a healthy discomfiture at being in a hospital and the awkwardness of being the new boyfriend while her folks- especially her mom- looked after her, talked to the doctors and nurses, and made care decisions. I saw dynamics and heard medical terminology that left me reeling and feeling helpless. It ultimately was an epiphany though for Erika, for her folks and for me.

Erika knew that we had a chance after that first surgery that I'd been a part of: I saw her at what she considered to be her worst and I stayed. She told me later that's when she knew I was the one. Her mom graciously offered me an out during that surgery, telling me that no one would blame me if it was too much or if I couldn't deal with it. While she was looking out for me on one level, of course it was all for Erika's sake. Anyone that sought a serious relationship with her daughter would be taking on all the hardship and worry that comes with a complex congenital heart condition and ultimately would be the one at Erika's bedside.

For my part, I can only write here what I told my mother-in-law then. You can't help who you fall in love with. Erika knew after the surgery that I was the one, but I knew before that. I saw what we would be up against. I realized I had much to learn and it would be a long time until I was the one holding her hand first, making care decisions with her, and understanding her situation and its ramifications. But I loved her, warts and all.

My folks asked me about it too, and of course I thought about it--who wouldn't? Love can be a force to motivate and bind, but you have to be pragmatic. If I wanted a family, could she? If we did, what were the chances the children could have the same problems? How long can she work? What does insurance cover? Will I get shocked if I'm near her? What would that be like? Can I handle seeing her as a patient? What would I do if the worst happened? These were my thoughts and my folks urged me to look at all of the angles, for my own good. They really liked her but they worried about their son as any parent would.

My dad told me much later that my response taught them something, though I didn't realize it at the time. I told them the same thing I told Erika's mom- you can't help who you fall in love with. I took it one step further with them, however, addressing the mortality considerations: Yes, she could be gone tomorrow but so could I, anyone could. It's said, that tomorrow is promised to no one and I agree. You can't live life worrying about it - that's not living. You have to take the risks with the rewards. I saw myself with Erika and that was a huge reward.

Along the way, I decided to discern whether I could share in Erika's Catholic faith. I had never really gone to church and while I had some Christian beliefs, religion was pretty much a complete mystery to me. I went through an R.C.I.A. (Rite of Christian Initiation for Adults) program and ultimately joined the Church to the delight of Erika and her family. Erika wanted a big Catholic wedding (not that we had a choice on the big part because she has a huge family and a million friends).

Most important to me though, was that this new faith taught me that we don't need to bear the challenges of life alone-- particularly the ones that faced us with Erika's situation. I learned that faith and prayer can help immeasurably and I'm forever thankful for that. I also recall a lesson that a nice couple shared with us as we went through pre-marriage counseling: Your marriage is a hope chest, to be filled with the good things you share. You only put things in it that make you stronger and closer as a couple. Nothing else goes in, you set that stuff aside. For me, that meant setting the anxiety aside and embracing life with Erika, for however long we're allowed to.

There was still the matter of starting a family. God, after all, wants us to be fruitful and multiply! We both wanted children, at least one. We consulted with a wonderful doctor who specialized in obstetrics for high-risk cardiac patients like Erika. He assured us he saw no reason we couldn't try, counseling us not to wait long, though. Soon after that discussion we married, bought a house, and learned we were having a baby. I still remember the day we told our folks, only 6 weeks in. We wanted to be up front with her pregnancy in case health concerns arose. It's a good thing we did but the day we announced it, it was a good day.

The bottom almost dropped from beneath us a couple months in. Erika was diagnosed with a partial placenta abruption. The doctor ordered significant bed-rest for something like six months. That shook me up, I worried both for our baby and Erika. I wondered if we'd made a mistake, if we shouldn't be doing this (my faith said trust in God). We worried about whether the baby would have a heart problem. Erika stayed home, able to do some work remotely and things stabilized. We went to many, many appointments and enjoyed many more ultrasounds than the usual anxious parents do. The baby was growing, moving, living. We decided against learning the sex since we wanted to have a nice surprise at the end, given the tension and anxiety we were going through.

The doctor kept telling us, we have to get to 27 weeks and then if the baby has to be born, it will have a good chance. We made it 33 weeks and Erika went into labor, 5 weeks early. The doctors tried to stop it but the labor continued. I worried so much, I barely slept. They didn't really want to do a C-section due to Erika's situation but she wasn't dilating much. After two and a half days of labor, the baby started to show signs of distress. The baby had to be delivered surgically.

Ethan Matthew was born, a tiny thing of 4 pounds, 4 ounces, with a headful of red hair. He cried a good healthy cry and his heart was good. His daddy's eyes overflowed with proud tears. I remember it seemed like thirty people were in the room; the whole floor wanted to know what we were having since it was rare not to know ahead of time. Once he came out, it seemed like half the people left. They weren't there just to find out if it was a he or she, were they?

Ethan's umbilical cord was as thin as a pencil and he'd have to spend a week in the N.I.C.U., but he would be fine. Much later, our doctor confessed he wasn't sure we were going to get a baby out of this. But here he was, a true miracle, and I'd never felt such euphoria. You did it, Erika, you did it. He's here and he's healthy. And, thank God, so was my wife. She just wanted to know if his heart was good, and it was. Thank God.

We were going to stop with Ethan, the whole situation scared us both. I find we consider Erika's situation when making certain decisions. Having kids was a huge concern. Deciding where to live was another. Prior to getting a house, we explored moving to Chicago. We would have been virtually alone, far from her doctors and family who made up an important support system for both of us. We both come from close-knit families and we decided it was best to stay close, especially since we wanted kids.

I learned about Erika's coping mechanisms as we went. We met others with ICDs and I learned how people with them avoid the particular situations that they were in when their defibrillator went off. For example, Erika told me about one fellow whose ICD went off when he took a shower in the morning, so he started showering at night. Based on what Erika's gone through, I can't blame them. Her biggest fear was always, "What if it goes off?" It's not just the pain. It's a complex weave of emotions, embarrassment, worry, fear, sadness, anger, and helplessness. Don't underestimate the pain though. I hear it's like getting kicked in the chest by a horse. ICDs save lives, but those with them definitely have a love-hate relationship with them. I personally love it, 110%. It keeps my wife at my side, where she belongs.

The closest I've been when Erika's ICD went off was in the middle of the night. We were sleeping and I swear I sensed it was coming just before it did, I don't know how. But I saw this brilliant flash of light prior to opening my eyes. What I think happened though was that the shock set off the static in the blankets, resulting in this relatively bright flash. I felt a bit of a static shock. She was OK but we found out that her ICD was giving unnecessary therapies- yet another trip to the E.R.

There have been many visits to the hospital. I think we can usually count on one visit a year, often for different things. Getting the ICD back in, problems with drug interactions, arrhythmias that weren't stopping, infections, and new ICDs. The scariest visit by far was when Erika needed a pulmonary valve implanted to help fend off further enlargement of her heart (left untreated, a very bad thing). That was the first open-heart surgery she'd had since I was with her and I was terrified. I relied heavily on both my family and hers to get us through. My clearest memory is when the doctor came in after a very, very long and anxious wait- to tell us that the surgery was a success and Erika was on her way to recovery. I remember collapsing shortly after, into a warm and much needed hug from my family.

Erika needs a support system, that's obvious, but spouses also need help. No one should bear this alone. A huge team of physicians, technicians, pharmacists and nurses look after Erika's well-being medically. She and I now make all of her care decisions. I know more about cardiology than I'd ever imagine wanting to know. I'm a hospital pro, now. Bring a book, wear layers (hospitals can be cold) and comfortable shoes. You wait, a lot. Seriously, hospitals are about the waiting and waiting and waiting some more.

One must come to terms with the fact that our medical professionals can't fix everything. They don't know everything. It's OK to question anything and everything. As Erika-the-patient's spouse I have to be her advocate, a detective, a bouncer, a listener, a complainer, an arguer, a liaison, a sounding board, and an inquisitor. It's OK to cry, to pray, to be angry and frustrated. It's okay to say nothing to your loved ones, just hold their hands, and just be there. Most importantly, when the crisis is over and you're back home, it's OK to slip back into a "normal" life, be a "normal" couple, and let the memory of the last incident fade.

Life went on for us after the valve surgery. We started camping, Erika had her gall bladder removed, and we had a surprise pregnancy. Yes, despite our intentions, we found out we were pregnant again. It went much better and this time we found out what we were having a little girl--daddy's girl who I call my little Jumping Bean because she had hiccups in the womb and would jump around during ultrasounds. We had the same worries about whether she'd have heart problems, and of course I worried about my wife. But Erika worked the whole time and was mostly fine until showing signs of congestive heart failure toward the 34th week. Our doctor said, "God made this decision easy." Sophie Catherine entered the world on a snowy Wednesday, another preemie but outweighing her brother by a pound (5 pounds, 4 ounces).

We're a typical family, but I thought early on that the kids need not be shielded from Erika's condition. They knew from an early age that she goes to the doctor often and has an "ouchie" heart that needs looking after. I wanted it all as just part of our lives, and so far it has worked well with the help of wonderful parents and families on both sides. They've been a huge part of our lives and we've leaned on them heavily.

We try to keep things "normal." Erika has said many times that she just wants to be 'normal'. To me, our lives are normal. I know what she means, and she's certainly entitled to her woe-is-me days. When she gets a shock (which is fortunately- knock on wood- a rare occurrence), she handles it pretty well now. But there is an inevitable delay and then she gets a bit morose and weepy a day or two after. When her heart goes willy-nilly (and not just because I enter the room), I can always tell because she kind of freezes, sits forward, raises her arm a bit like she's going to make a muscle, and clenches that fist. Sometimes she counts her pulse- counting beats is a big part of getting through an event. And I have to talk to her, about anything, which is tough because I'm not much of a small-talker. That drives Erika nuts. See, we're just another average married couple!

I'm still not always sure how to act or what to say when something's happening. Erika has atrial fibrillation now. While it's not as bad as ventricular tachycardia, it is still scary because clots can form and clots are bad--potentially scary-bad. So when an event happens, sometimes it can last hours and we have to weigh going to the ER. I catch myself thinking about her condition when making travel plans, too. For instance, I'd love to go to Yellowstone with the family and go hiking out there, but is that wise given what could happen? How fast could we get to a hospital? Is there a good one nearby?

Mostly though, we just take things as they come. For me, as a spouse, things are pretty normal. I don't think about her condition daily, like she does. She has to, it's always there. She suffers little runs of arrhythmias, moments of light-headedness, little reminders of mortality, and of how fragile this all is. But we don't let it dictate life to us. We live the best we can, we have fun, we raise our children and we enjoy our family and friends. We live in the present, with a cautious eye on the future. We live.

Do I have any regrets? I have more wishes than regrets. I wish Erika didn't have a congenital heart condition. I wish I always knew the right thing to say or do. I wish Erika didn't need the ICD, didn't have the worry, and didn't have to go through those surgeries. But this is all a part of her, a part of her life and therefore it's all part of my life, a part of me. It's made her the person she is: a loving mom, a successful professional, a dedicated advocate, and a strong survivor. Most importantly to me, it's made her the wife and companion I was meant to have and will always cherish, whatever may come. I'll never regret it.

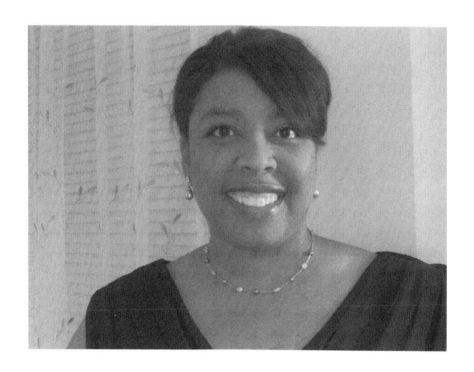

CHAPTER 5: YES, I'D LIKE TO USE ONE OF MY LIFELINES!

Phyllis

I imagine it was like a scene out of the TV show, *ER* with bells sounding and buzzers chirping, nurses and doctors running down the hall, holding their stethoscopes, white coats flapping. As I lay watching Saturday Night Live, I heard the loud slapping of their feet pounding the hallway floor and wondered who they were running to attend to. When they burst into my room, I realized it was me!

It was a Saturday night in March and I was in the cardiac ward of the University of Michigan hospital. At 36, I was probably the youngest patient on the floor. I was into the second weekend of my stay and figured I must be pretty sick because I had been there for almost two weeks and they still didn't know what was wrong with me. Lying in my bed, watching some silly comedy skit, I was unaware that my heart rate had skyrocketed within a matter of seconds. But the monitors had seen it and that's what sent those docs and nurses bearing down on my room.

John, the resident, burst in first and snapped on the light, his eyes wide and wild as he ran to my bed. He was followed by two or three other nurses and they all surrounded me. First they looked up at the monitors and then down at me. Up then down. Up then down again. Something wasn't right. Then finally John said, "Hey, how are you doing?" Although I answered fine, it was obvious something wasn't fine since the cavalry was in my room. The monitors at the nurse's station had said my pulse was somewhere around 280, which had sent them racing to my room. They checked my pulse manually, first at my wrist, then at my neck. But just like that, my heart rate was back to normal.

Before that night in 2006, I really hadn't given too much thought to my heart rate. Like others, I would stop and check my pulse when my step aerobics instructor told us to. Often mine would be on the high end of the scale he suggested, but since I didn't feel bad or sick, I just chalked it up to my joy of exercising.

Years earlier I had started working out, mainly as a way to escape from my job as a college residence hall director. At first I just liked being off campus and hanging out with "grownups." But after a while, I found I really enjoyed exercising. Step aerobic classes, kickboxing, balance boards, Pilates—if it was new and different, I wanted to try it. After six years being active, I had lost about 50 pounds, three dress sizes and countless inches. I was in the best shape of my life. Then in 2005, that all changed.

Due to a condition unrelated to my heart, I had a surgery that kept me bed-bound in the hospital for over a month. After a two month recovery to get myself back to walking again, I resumed my usual exercise activities. However, I found myself getting more winded earlier in my workouts and at night, I could hear a "gurgling" in my chest when I laid down to sleep. At a normal follow-up appointment with my surgeon, I shared my concerns. He noticed my heart rate was fast and abnormal, but didn't believe it had anything to do with the surgery they had recently performed. He suggested that I follow-up with my primary care physician.

My PCP arranged for me to see a cardiologist who specialized in ICDs. After running some tests, he saw that I had an arrhythmia but he didn't know why. He then noted that it was very likely that I would eventually need an ICD to protect myself from a sudden arrhythmia that might be fatal. I may have heard about arrhythmias before, but this was certainly the first time I ever heard of ICDs. I questioned why I should get this device, if he didn't know why I had arrhythmias. Although he did explain the procedure, the device, what it could do and why I needed it, I didn't get the impression that getting one was something I immediately needed to do. I could decide to get an ICD or not.

I left that appointment not ever expecting to have to make that decision. I fell back into my normal routine and began seeing Dr. Dyke, who would become my primary cardiologist. He put me on a regimen of anti-arrhythmia drugs and took a "wait and see" approach, monitoring me for about 6 months while he tried to figure out what was wrong with my heart. During this time, I had an opportunity to go with my sister to Orlando for her company's annual conference. With Disney World and Universal Studios just down the road, I was excited to go, as both of us are amusement park and roller coaster junkies. I asked for Dr. Dyke's blessing. He gave it, but instructed me to stick to land-based rides and forego the roller coasters.

Not ride rollers coasters! Was he insane?! I had been riding coasters since my head first cleared the height limit. Visiting the amusement park Cedar Point in Sandusky, Ohio was a hallowed family tradition each summer, sometimes twice. Forget the merry-go-rounds and ferris wheels, we were roller coaster girls. So much so, that my sister and I would joke that we'd be two old ladies with grey hair, in line for the latest and greatest coaster. We'd never stop.

July 19, 2005. That was the day I rode my last roller coaster— twice. We had stayed two extra days after the conference and giddily strapped ourselves into the Spiderman ride at Universal Studios Island of Adventures. Technically it was not a roller coaster, since it doesn't leave the ground. It does, however, include a virtual 400 foot freefall experience. I did not know this.

Normally, I could vividly recall the details of almost any ride. This one is a blur. Sitting next to my sister, who kept pointing out little things for me to see, I had started sweating. I'm not a big sweater, so I knew something was a little off. My heart pounded quicker and it began to get hot in the ride. Even with the scant four minute length, I was ready for it to be over. When it came time for the freefall, I closed my eyes. This was the first time—ever—I had closed my eyes on the descent, the best part of the ride. Afterwards, we'd normally chat excitedly about what we liked best and replay the experience in our minds. This time, I just wanted to sit down and feel the breeze (in Orlando?!) on my face. I felt jittery and it was hard to breathe in the stifling humidity.

Unaware of the distress I was concealing, my sister went off to ride the Incredible Hulk roller coaster. While she was gone, I calmed myself down and talked myself out of thinking I just had an arrhythmia. Of course, now I know I did. Even so, I sat with jealousy watching my sister scream her lungs out as she experienced weightless zero g's and barrel rolls on the Incredible Hulk coaster. I wanted to again feel the rush and excitement and lamented the fact that I probably never would. After her coaster ride, my sister was on a high and eagerly asked if I wanted to ride the Spiderman again. I think she sensed my sadness and wanted to cheer me up.

Part of me didn't want to go through that dizzy feeling again. But not wanting to show any weakness—after all this was my comrade in coasters—I said yes. This time, I closed my eyes through the whole ride. I knew then that this part of my life was over. No more Cedar Point, which held countless memories of family fun. No more dreams of riding roller coasters well into my 50's. No more "sisters only" vacations centered around amusement parks. I spent the next day and a half riding grandma friendly things like "Dumbo" and "Cat in the Hat." Boring.

Summer ended and Dr. Dyke continued to schedule me for tests to confirm or rule out possibilities for my arrhythmias. I can no longer remember all the tests I did but sometimes, in medicine, figuring out what the problem is takes a lot of figuring out what it's not. So, I had been giving my same story to everyone who walked in the door. And, that was a lot of people. They all wanted to test their theories.

Was it an infection? No. Was it a heart attack? No. Was it related to my other elusive cellular condition? No.

Finally something started pointing Dr. Dyke in the direction of a condition called sarcoidosis. I now know sarcoidosis as the disease that contributed to the death of comedian Bernie Mac and professional footballer Reggie White, but at that time I had never heard of it. Sarcoidosis is a disease in which abnormal collections of chronic inflammatory cells, aka granulomas, form as nodules in multiple organs, particularly the lungs and lymph nodes. Lung scarring or infection may lead to respiratory failure and death. The majority of sarcoidosis sufferers have the lung version.

However, I am not normal. I have cardiac sarcoidosis. Of course I would have to have one of the more rare versions. Symptoms can range from conduction abnormalities to fatal ventricular arrhythmias. I've read that, although cardiac involvement is present in about 20-30% of sarcoid patients, only about 5% are symptomatic, like me. Similar to Reggie White, I could suffer a fatal arrhythmia which could lead to my death.

Having a name to what's wrong with me didn't necessarily make it easier to accept. Especially since not much is known about why people, especially African American females, get sarcoidosis. But I began reading up on the disease, getting a crash course on the inner workings of the heart. Terms like V-tach and V-fib became part of my everyday vocabulary. Even so, it took a simple story of a train on a railroad track to put into perspective what was happening to my heart. This is the story, as close as I can remember:

"Your hearts primary function is to pump the blood through your body, giving you life. Electrical impulses tell your heart to contract, or as you might say, beat. Now imagine the electrical impulses as a train and the train tracks are what the electrical impulses follow in order to get to its destination, which is where your heart beats, or Beatsville! In a normal heart, the train follows the shortest, most direct route to Beatsville. Remember those old silent movies where the villain lays his hostage across the train tracks to stop the train and rob it? That hostage on the train tracks is the sarcoid granulomas on your heart's electrical tracks, which can impede the train from reaching Beatsville (in a timely manner or even, ever). This causes the train—the electrical impulses—to have to jump the track. In the worst case scenario, the train stops. But in your case, your train jumps to another track, running out of control and now you have a runaway train, or an arrhythmia. You need an ICD to stop the train from jumping the track and running out of control." A simple story but it made sense.

Dr. Dyke continued scheduling me for tests to try and figure out where exactly the sarcoid was located on my heart. The thought was that if they could remove the sarcoid granulomas, or that hostage lying across my electrical tracks, they could stop the arrhythmias. They biopsied a part of my heart, but the part they biopsied didn't have the sarcoid and they couldn't locate it. So he ordered a procedure called an ablation. In its simplest form, an ablation is the removal of material from the surface of an object by vaporization, chipping or other erosive processes (source, Wikipedia). Say what?!? I remember once some kids had spray painted the side of my high school and a company came out and essentially did an ablation by sandblasting the graffiti away. So, that was what they were going to do to my heart!

Seriously though, non-surgical ablation, used for many types of arrhythmias, is performed in a special lab called the electrophysiology (EP) laboratory. During this non-surgical procedure a catheter is inserted into a specific area of the heart. A special machine directs energy through the catheter to small areas of the heart muscle that causes the abnormal heart rhythm. This energy "disconnects" the source of the abnormal rhythm from the rest of the heart (source, WebMD). It would have been sweet, if it had worked. But it didn't. And a few months later, my train jumped the track.

It was a normal work day and I was trying to finish up a project before the end of the day. I stood up at my desk to go to the bathroom and immediately got dizzy. I stood there for a moment or two and held on to the desk to stop the room from spinning. One of my co-workers happened past my office at that exact moment. She was shocked to see my face was white as a sheet and ashen. She helped me sit down and brought me a glass of water.

Trying to stop her fussing, I said I was okay but she kept telling me I didn't look okay. Luckily my PCP's office was right across the street in the student health center, so I went over to get a walk-in appointment. Upon running an electrocardiogram, my PCP ordered me to go directly to the University hospital. Do not pass go, she said. She had called ahead and they were expecting me in the ER. She wouldn't even allow me to drive myself, even though the hospital was just a few blocks away. I would later find out that I had third degree heart block. Oh boy!

So it was here, at the University of Michigan hospital, that I stayed for about two weeks as they tried to figure out what to do next. A parade of doctors, nurses and specialists descended on my room. However, I was an exemplary patient, never grousing about the tests I was scheduled for, only requiring that anyone who wanted to enter my room to introduce their self and the reason for their visit—had to do it in layman terms. I told them if they couldn't make me understand it, they weren't good doctors! It was the only way I could keep from feeling like a human lab specimen.

I became quite the celebrity, since I was always up and had my "face" on at 6am, cracking jokes with the residents as they made their morning rounds. Many doctors and residents would stop by just to say hi and to follow my case, even if they weren't assigned to me. It was a fun room because I never had my TV droning on, like the other patients. Since I worked every day, I had no interest in watching Maury Povich (You are not the father!) or the People's Court. My radio was always tuned to the local R&B station, a party just waiting for some party-goers. The staff teased that I was the only patient on the floor who always had at least one visitor a day.

Although it was kinda fun being in the hospital, it really wasn't until that fateful Saturday night, watching Saturday Night Live and having my heart rate skyrocket, did the full weight of my condition come crashing down on me. After the ruckus died down that night and the staff left my room, John, my favorite resident, retuned to check on me. We sat in my darken room—me lying in bed, John perched at the window—and reviewed what had happened. Since I hadn't really felt anything, I kept telling myself it wasn't so bad; John thought otherwise. He reached out to my hand, concern lacing his words.

He explained how sudden my heart rate could elevate and subside. Because of that, he wanted to move me to the Cardiac Intensive Care unit in the hospital. Here I would be closely monitored and have a staff member right outside my door, just in case. He also wanted to consult with a cardiologist who specialized in ICDs. He felt strongly that I needed one now.

The next morning, I was moved to the ICU and was to stay there until my scheduled ICD implantation, which was three days away. Even after talking further with the specialists about ICDs, I still wasn't too keen on getting this device but kept remembering John's concerned voice from the previous night. As I think back, it really was his concern that made the difference. Of course, as a doctor, he would present all the options for me to make an informed decision to protect myself. But he spoke to me that night as a friend and it really touched me. In addition, the other residents all came by after they heard I had been moved and they too shared their concern for me.

March 6, 2006. I was not mentally prepared when they told me I was scheduled a day early to get my ICD. What?! But no one was around. It was a Monday, all my friends were working and, wouldn't you know it, not a soul came to visit me that day (My parents were deferring their visit until the next day to be around for the surgery). I couldn't get anyone on the phone and was trying hard not to flip out and leave weird "my-life-is-passing-in-front-of-my-eyes" messages on my sister's and parent's answering machines. I had begun to panic, thinking I couldn't go into surgery without seeing or at least talking to my parents, when my mom finally called. She tried to calm me down by phone but it just wasn't the same. We prayed together, then hung up.

While I laid there staring up at the ceiling, waiting for them to wheel me away, the oddest person walked into my room. It was a Catholic priest, looking for the previous occupant of my room (who I knew had unfortunately passed away). I tentatively asked if the priest would pray with me, even though I was Lutheran. He chuckled and said we were all sisters and brothers in Christ. He began praying. Hearing the similar words of his prayer, I felt a sudden calmness and knew everything would work out all right. Now I understand the saying, "He might not come when you want him, but God is always right on time." Amen!

Waking up, it was still hard to believe I had something implanted near my heart. Well, that was until I tried to lift my left arm. Oh, the pain. The next few days were a blur and I couldn't keep anything down because of the anesthesia. But I still managed to wake up for the morning rounds to talk and joke with the residents. That was the best part of my day.

The rest of the day I began to grow more and more concerned about my heart rate, sometimes staring at the monitor for minutes on end watching my heart rate increase (oh no!) or subside (phew!). The doctors had conservatively set the upper limit of my ICD at 150, which is pretty low, to protect me from the arrhythmias they couldn't predict. Afraid I might increase my heart rate to the point of shocking myself, I rarely got up from my bed or walked around my room. I even stopped laughing. The doctors began to worry about me. John and the other residents tried to cheer me up, one even made me a cd of songs that he knew I liked. Each day they'd talk to me about how the ICD was there to protect me and that I shouldn't be afraid to live.

Leaving the hospital a few days later, with my left arm in a sling, should have been a celebration. Instead, it was the scariest things I'd ever done in my life. I had been in the hospital for over three weeks, protected by scores of people around who knew me and were trained to help me, if anything were to go wrong. Walking from the car to my apartment, I was very aware of everything going on in my body and attuned to every little thing. I secretly kept checking my pulse at my wrist or neck. If my heart started beating faster, I was concerned. If it skipped a beat, I was concerned. If it beat correctly, I was concerned.

That night, I tried to get a comfortable position in bed. I couldn't lie on my back, because it hurt my shoulder lying flat. I couldn't lie on my preferred left side because of the sling. In addition, on my left side, I could hear my heart beating against the mattress. Imagine listening to your heart beat—beat—beat—skipped beat—beat! That just didn't work. I stayed awake all night, getting only a few minutes of sleep.

My sister had driven in from Pittsburgh to stay with me for the week. When it came time for her to go, I cried. I didn't want to be alone. What if something happened? What would I do if I got a shock? For my peace of mind, I ordered the Lifeline systems for use in my apartment. Yes, at 36, I wore a button similar to that silly commercial, "Help I've fallen and I can't get up." I didn't care how stupid it sounded or looked. Actually, the "pendant" is quite fashionable—NOT! But I felt safe. In my apartment, that is. Out in the world was another story.

I was convinced I could control whether or not I got a shock. My theory? Don't do anything to raise my heart rate! I began wearing my exercise heart rate monitor all the time. To keep my heart rate down, I would walk very slow everywhere I went. I avoided stairs and inclines. It got so bad that before agreeing to go somewhere, I had to research the environment. What floor was it on? Was there an elevator? How far was the elevator from the entrance/exit? A lot of things needed to fall into place for me to feel okay about venturing out.

Afraid of getting a shock while driving, I convinced the hospital social worker to "prescribe" me a discount ADA (**Americans with Disabilities Act**) pass for the city bus & cab system. With this pass, I got reduced cab rides to and from any medical appointments or rides to take care of things like grocery shopping or errands. Sometimes we'd have to stop and pick up other riders, making a short trip to the doctor's office take several hours instead of 60 minutes. But I didn't care, as long as someone else was around to help me, should I need it. I didn't like being alone.

There was no one around the first time I got shocked. Tired of watching my waistline expand (due to medications & inactivity), I tried to get back into my workout routine. Staff at the Cardiac Rehab Center had suggested I start with 15 minutes of walking on the treadmill on the days I didn't attend Phase I rehab classes. Treadmill, really?!? I was used to complicated step aerobics routines and kickboxing not a boring treadmill, but I was willing to give it a go. Pre-ICD I had been a daily fixture in my apartment's exercise room, regularly bringing my aerobic step and video tapes to play in the VCR or my sparring gloves for kickboxing. So one day after dinner, I decided to walk myself over to the clubhouse, which was about 350 feet away from the building I lived in, and do my 15 minutes on the treadmill. All my life I had counted things to occupy my mind, so yes, I knew it took about 350 steps to get to the clubhouse. Weird, I know!

Before leaving I called my mom to let her know where I was going. She knew how distraught I was with my weight gain and I groused with her about just how effective could 15 minutes really be in peeling off the pounds. Normally I would exercise for at least an hour each day after work, and there would be 2 or 3 other residents in the clubhouse. But at 7:00 pm, there was no one else around and, even though there was a security camera in the room, no one was monitoring it since the leasing office was closed.

It all happened so quickly. I stepped on the belt and started the treadmill going, slowly beginning to walk. I guess my heart rate had been a little elevated from the walk over, because when I casually looked down at the monitor on my wrist a few minutes later, it read 148. 148!?! If accurate, that was only 2 points away from the dreaded 150. And I knew my monitor was accurate, as I had calibrated it with the high tech monitors they used at Cardiac Rehab. I quickly sat down on the nearest thing I could find, a recumbent exercise bike, and tried to control my heart rate through breathing. No dice. Since I was just short of flipping out, deep breathing was not going to stop it. It now read 158. I braced for the shock I knew was coming.

Boom! The first time is really not that bad. Since you have nothing to compare it with, it's just something that happens and you experience it with a little bit of awe tinged with fear. Everyone always wants to know what it feels like. There is really no way to accurately describe it. I guess if I had to, I'd say it feels like a very large firecracker went off in your chest. You can feel it deep in your chest as your heart knocks against, what I imagine, is your rib cage. I'm not sure if it makes a sound that others can hear, but I could hear it. It sounded like a deep, booming clap of thunder that comes out of the blue and startles you, no matter what you're doing. The scariest part is not knowing when it's going to happen.

But I had my heart rate monitor on, so I knew that it was going to happen. And, I could see that my heart rate was not subsiding, so I knew it was going to happen again. Boom! Slowly my heart rate started to decrease. I sat there frantically searching my mind trying to figure out what to do. Then it came to me. Even though I had my bulky cell phone (remember this is 2006!), I didn't know the address to the clubhouse and I didn't think I could go through explaining what was happening to some random person at 911. In my mind, I needed to get to the safest place I knew—my apartment. I needed my Lifeline. So I began the walk home.

I made it out of the clubhouse and down the pathway before getting shocked again. That was #3. In my mind, I just keep repeating, "I need Lifeline"…20 steps…Boom!…"I need Lifeline"…20 more steps…Boom! Thinking back, I'm not sure how I managed to stay on my feet. I guess it was my single-minded determination that kept me going. I needed my Lifeline.

Finally, by counting my steps, I reached the door to my apartment building. Boom! Another shock. Once inside I quickly pressed the Lifeline button around my neck, knowing that Lifeline would send an ambulance even if I couldn't verbally respond. Thankfully, I lived on the first floor, because I'm not sure I physically could have handled climbing a flight of stairs. With uncannily steady hands, I used my key to open the door to my apartment. Boom! I walked directly to the Lifeline transmitter I kept in the dining room next to the wall phone. I clumsily sat down at my glass topped dining room table, just as my Lifeline call connected. "Phyllis, this is Lifeline. Do you need help?" I turned to the transmitter as if it were an actual person and said, "Yes, I'm getting shocked. I need help now." The representative sprang into action, first calling for an ambulance and then starting to call my emergency phone tree.

When you first subscribe to Lifeline, you set up a list of people who should be called for you in case of an emergency—your first responders. These should be people who can get to you relatively quickly and have access to your residence. Luckily a few weeks earlier I had stepped out on faith and asked my upstairs neighbors (a couple who I had only talked to in passing) to be my first responders and had given them a key to my apartment (talk about faith indeed!). After receiving the call, my neighbor rushed right down, with her eight month old baby in her arms. Even though she had a key, she courteously knocked at my door before realizing I had accidently left it ajar. She sat down at the table and after confirming an ambulance was on the way, just held my hand. Just having her there made a world of difference. However, my heart rate continued to be elevated, and each time I got a shock I would let out a short scream, like a hiccup. The baby thought it was a game and she joined in, eerily synchronizing her shouts with mine.

Where I live, the local fire department is the first response team. So a few minutes later, in walk two guys in full fireman gear! (This story just keeps getting better and better!) After making sure I was not on fire, they took my vitals and wanted to get me up on the stretcher for the arrival of the ambulance. But every time I tried to get on the stretcher I got a shock, so I stubbornly refused to move. The ambulance arrived and I still refused. All this time, my connection to Lifeline was still active and the rep could hear everything that was happening. With me connected to Lifeline, my mom had been trying to get through on the phone but couldn't. She called Lifeline directly. The rep briefed my mother and then patched her through the Lifeline transmitter.

Out of the blue I hear, "Phyllis Arlene, this is your mother. Get up on that stretcher so these good people can help you!" Well, that did it. Her voice brooked no refusal. I dare you to tell me what adult, when hearing their full name called out by their mother, would not comply. She meant business. I got on the stretcher, receiving a shock for my efforts. They wheeled me to the ambulance and then drove to the hospital, where I stayed for several days. When it was all said and done, I had received a total of 11 shocks. Wisely, the doctors raised the limit on my ICD to 178, instead of 150. Hallelujah!

I wish I could tell you that I never was shocked again. Unfortunately I developed a real panic driven aversion to shocking. I believe I had at least 2, maybe 3, more incidents of shocking that year that led me to the hospital. I do know that one time, the shock was due to an actual arrhythmia, but the other times were all anxiety-based. I began avoiding locations I had been shocked in, which included my shower. I became so afraid to shower, that I convinced the hospital social worker I needed help bathing (as you can see, I'm a pretty persuasive woman!). She "prescribed" a bathing assistant to come to my house every other day. She would stand in the bathroom, while I showered with the curtain half open—oh boy, did water spill everywhere! Everyone was sympathetic, but I could tell they were starting to get fed up with me. And so was I.

My PCP recommended a therapist to help me cope. So twice a week, I'd take an ADA cab(!) over to see this guy and we'd talk about all sorts of things, including my fears of being shocked. There were lots of tears and lots of grieving for my former self. I truly believe it helped, and after a while I told myself to snap out of this funk that I was in. And really, I think that's what did it. I had just had enough. Enough of feeling sorry for myself. Enough of being scared. Enough of being always on alert. Everyone, I reasoned, had something wrong with them. Mine just happened to be a really weird thing that I couldn't control. Deal with it!   And, so I played the hand I was dealt.

I went back to work and started driving again. I rearranged my work schedule to allow me to exercise at the Cardiac Rehab Center. I would attend Phase III, which is like a health club for patients who are no longer participating in the mandatory rehab classes. There are treadmills, elliptical machines, bikes, weight machines, free weights, swiss balls, and a cardio room complete with a dance floor, music and a wall-to-wall mirror—basically anything you'd find in a health club. But with the added benefit of exercise physiologists and nurses to respond if anything were to happen. After you arrive, they take your blood pressure and chart your weight, then off you go. You are free to do your own thing, or if you ask, any staff member will work out with you. They'll even check your heart rate intermittently, if you don't have your own monitor.

Since I knew all the staff and interns, it was a comfortable place to work out. My favorite machine to use was the elliptical. But one day all three were taken, so I decided to tackle my old nemesis—the treadmill. Just thinking of getting on that thing caused panic. So I asked one of the exercise physiologists, who knew my history with treadmills well, if he would just walk on the treadmill next to me and talk while we both walked. The first time, I was still so scared that I didn't really participate in the conversation because that, of course, would raise my heart rate. So he just talked to me about what was happening in his life. The next few times got better and after about 4 times, I was able to get on the treadmill sans a chaperone.

Unfortunately, the Cardiac Rehab Center doesn't have health club hours and it closes at 6 pm. Normally, I'd leave my office at 4:30 on the dot, and drive the few miles to Domino Farms where Phase

III is located, getting there by 4:45. I'd have at least 1 hour to get in a good workout. However recently, because of afterhours work events and new responsibilities helping my mom, I had been unable to get in during those limited times. Frustrated that I was missing my workouts, I decided to buy an elliptical machine for my home use. I have recently bought a house and turned the room designated as an office, into an exercise room instead. And, of course, I have Lifeline in my new house.

If this were a made-for-TV movie, this would be the part where the actress playing me would show how I've overcome adversity by running a 15K marathon or climbing a snow-capped mountain, standing at the top shouting, "Drago" like Sylvester Stallone in that *Rocky* movie. But it's not and, no story can be neatly wrapped up with a pretty little bow. Yes, I still have my freak out moments, here and there. Yes, I still take a boat load of pills to control my arrhythmias. But there are good things too. Like last fall, I started ballroom dancing lessons. I'll admit that the first few times I wore my heart rate monitor (just to get a feel for things, thank you), but now I'm practically old salt at it, and I know when to put on the steam and when to pull it back some. And, since I wear black & white swing shoes with the ribbon laces tied in neat bows, I guess things *can* be wrapped up nicely!

With the exception of one appropriate shock in January of 2008, I have been shock free for five years. I have had the battery replaced once in my ICD and continue to see Dr. Dyke on a quarterly basis. In addition, I have the pleasure of seeing the always amusing, Dr. Sisson on a bi-annual basis. He's my pulmonologist and teases me unrelentingly about my love life! Between my three doctors, I'm lucky to have this pretty amazing medical team looking out for me.

When Helen at the Device Clinic first called to ask me to write this chapter, I didn't call her back. It has been six years since I received my ICD and, even though I had spoken on a panel a few years ago at the annual ICD conference for young adults, I really didn't want to go through remembering all the things that had happened to me and trying to get them down on paper. But a week later, I was attending a conference about diversity, when one of the speakers said something that made me pause. He said, "Everyone has a story to tell and everyone's story should be told." So here's my story. I've told it. I don't necessarily feel any better or any worse. But I wanted to write this chapter to help others know that there is someone else out here that has experienced what they're going through and is still standing. I'm still standing and laughing and loving and crying and dancing and exercising and living, with my ICD. So when Helen called the second time, I answered the phone.

This chapter is lovingly dedicated to my father, Raymond (1932-2011) and mother, Gladys (1937-2012).

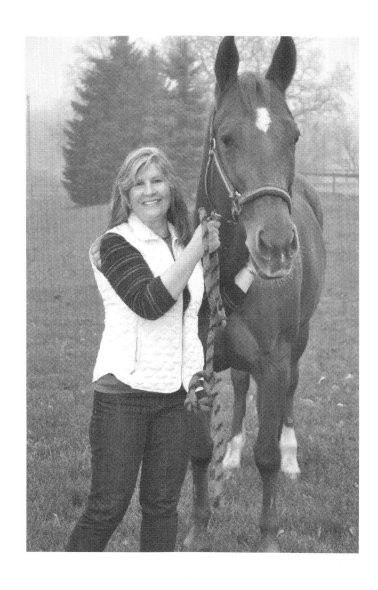

CHAPTER 6: LIVE YOUR DREAMS...ONE BEAT AT A TIME

Terri

Becoming part of the YOUNG ICD CONNECTION is a lot more exciting than receiving a very different invitation, to become part of AARP. I was invited to join that club because I just turned 55. Some people say that I do not look my age, but I will let you be the judge by my picture in this publication. (Please be kind!)

I have known my whole life that I have a complex congenital heart condition and have recently learned that I am one of the oldest surviving persons with that condition in Michigan. Whether you have recently learned of your heart condition, have known your entire life, or have a loved one or friend with heart abnormalities, we are all, in some way, connected. The reason for this connection is my friend and yours, the implantable cardioverter-defibrillator (ICD). I received my little ICD friend almost 3 years ago and will tell you about it in the next few pages.

Many of you have never met a heart patient older than yourself, so let me introduce myself – my name is Terri and I am living proof that you can live with an uncorrected congenital heart problem and still enjoy a good life. My heart condition consists of a ventricular septal defect (VSD), Pulmonary Stenosis (narrowing in the Pulmonary Artery), and L-transposition of the Great Arteries (LTGA). My diagnosis at birth was that I was a "blue baby" due to my lack of oxygen. I can only imagine the horror my parents felt when they learned that their baby, in the doctor's words, "probably would not live to adolescence".

Back in 1956, when I was born, survival with such conditions was virtually unheard of because surgical intervention was rarely considered, due to the medical knowledge and technology of the times. Thank God for Drs. Alfred Blaylock and Vivian Thomas, who pioneered the first open heart surgery on a "blue baby" at John's Hopkins Hospital. (Their collaboration was wonderfully portrayed in the movie Something the Lord Made.) The techniques they developed were later taught to other surgeons, including my heart surgeon, Dr. Herbert Sloan at University of Michigan Hospital. In 1960, Dr. Sloan performed that surgery on my heart, allowing me to be less cyanotic (blue) by opening up arteries and allowing additional oxygen into my system. Back then, the odds were not good, but by the grace of God, and the steady hands of my surgeons, plus the continuous support and compassion of my caregivers and family, I defied those odds. That surgery, at four years of age, gave me another chance at life. The other defects are still present. Sometimes I smile and think of my heart as driving on a highway in England; it seems backwards--"quite so," as they say over there - but it works! ☺

Going through life with congenital heart disease is challenging, limiting and is not an easy feat; but with hard work and a daily commitment to, as well as encouragement from my parents to stay as active and positive as possible, I turned my limitations into my own personal adventure—one that comes with challenges, as all adventures do. It is difficult to sum up 55 years of life into a few pages, but I will try by giving a few good examples.

When I was in elementary school, I was teased a lot-- especially by the boys. (Maybe they just liked me-- you know how boys are at that age!) Sometimes they were relentless in teasing me about my inability to take part in gym class, participate in outside activities in the cold, or even walk to school in the winter months. So, I tried to turn that situation around by telling them if they did not leave me alone, I would "give them my heart condition." As you can imagine, this was not a good idea, because now they were afraid of me. I felt like an outcast but I also chuckled at the thought that the boys would actually think I could do that. Boys!

No small child should need to know words like cyanosis, PVCs, and arrhythmias. We shouldn't hide from the truth, and my mother taught me the meaning of these words to help me understand why I could not do all the things the other kids could do. I began to connect these words to how I was feeling. For example, connecting the word cyanosis with being blue in color went along with the feeling of fatigue. Feeling blue. Understanding is a wonderful thing.

Camping, hiking, and skiing were activities that were off limits to me. My brother and sister were able to participate, but it was merely a dream for me. So, I used that time to read, which ultimately allowed me to get through school with high grades. I completed my Business degree at 19 and earned a degree in Veterinary Medicine at 45, the field in which I am currently employed. I am also completing classes to combine those two degrees into a bachelor's degree in Business Health. I believe you are never too old for education, as it is a lifelong pursuit.

As a child and teenager, I had problems riding a bicycle, especially on gravel. It was hard for me and very strenuous. So I learned how to ride a motorcycle. What a wonderful feeling that was, and still is, as I ride a 750cc Honda Shadow. I ride mostly with my younger brother, as he is my protector, and we have great times in the sun. The wind in your hair and the feeling of freedom is unlike any other. (Bugs in your face are not fun, however, so wear a helmet with a shield!)

The inability to participate in sports such as volleyball, basketball and track did not slow me down. I learned the fine art of cheerleading. Of course, it was different back then but cheerleading nonetheless. At first I became an alternate cheerleader, but the next year I was accepted on the team. Even now, I am one of the biggest cheerleaders of all! I cheer for my grandbabies (yes, my grandbabies – all five of them) sporting events as well as the Detroit Lions--for whom, by the way, I have waited 55+ years to become contenders. Go Lions and go grandbabies!

When I was first married, I was advised by my cardiologists that it would be risky to have a child. I am not saying that you should not listen to your doctor on this one, as all cases are different. In my case, when I became pregnant, the doctors quickly concluded that my baby and I would only have a 50% chance of survival. I decided that I would take the 50% chance and have the baby. I had a bouncing baby girl of 4 lbs 10 oz. and 19 inches long on a mild October evening. For me, it worked out wonderful. I was and am a "mommy," with immeasurable responsibilities and pride! My daughter Rebecca is healthy, happy and 33 years old at this writing. (I am certain she would try to tell you she is only in her 20s, but don't let her fool you!) I was able to raise my daughter just like any other mother. I worked outside the home, as so many of us do, but still had time and energy to help Rebecca with her homework. I taught her so many things in life and encouraged her to be the best she could be. I'll admit I lived vicariously through her at times, as I watched her extra-curricular activities in her cheerleading and pompon days. (She teases me in a good-natured way about my days as a cheerleading "alternate.") I always tried to keep her grounded and focused on school and family. At one point, we attended college together; and both received licensure in Veterinary Technology. In truth, my best friend was born that day in October. How many people can say this?

Running was never an option for me. So I learned to ride a horse in my preteen years. This was always a dream of mine and my cardiologist was in agreement with this decision—with one condition. If I ever fell off, he said I must sell the horse. Now anyone will tell you that learning to ride a horse has its ups and downs. I had a few small "downs" which I failed to mention to my cardiologist. ("My bad" as the kids of today would probably say.) In my 30s, I began learning English riding and jumping. I began with 10-15 minute lessons and worked my way up to 1-2 hour lessons, 4 days per week. I joined the MHJA (Michigan Hunter Jumper Association) and began jumping fences in competition along with my daughter. I can only tell you that it was one of the most rewarding experiences of my life.

Not only did I stay in perfect shape, but won Michigan's 1992 Championship in Primary Adult Jumping. (The same year, my daughter Rebecca won Reserve Champion in the state. I guess the apple doesn't fall far from the tree!) It is a thrill I will never forget, jumping 2-3 foot fences felt like I was flying through the air! Even with a severe complex congenital heart problem, I won the Championship against all the healthy hearts.   I think I took the lifelong practice of learning my limitations and dealing with them to a new level. And so can you!

On the subject of being a grandmother, I can only say it is the greatest! I have four grandsons and one granddaughter, they all call me Nana and I love them all so dearly that I cannot even begin to tell you.   Maybe I cannot keep up physically with "normal hearted" grandmas, but it doesn't matter! They love me just the same. I am always there for them and try to keep up as best as I can. This year alone, I have been involved in their soccer, football, special person's day, and even volunteered at their schools on occasion. Plus, I take them swimming, skiing (yes, I am learning to downhill ski on the bunny hill), golfing and to the fair. I must look a sight "trotting" down the sidelines screaming cheers of joy when one of my babies gets a goal, scores a touchdown, or putts the ball into the cup. Being a grandma is truly the BEST! It keeps you young and I would not miss one day with my babies!

April 3, 2009

Sitting in a café eating dinner after a long Friday at work was a good way to wind down. The work week had been a long one, filled with emergency cases, radiographs, cranky dogs and cats, plus a technician who was not feeling well. Dinner came and went and I felt much too full for dessert... when all of a sudden – lights out!

As I opened my eyes a bit dazed and confused, I looked around the room and realized I was lying in a hospital bed. The next thing I recognized were some I.V. lines, an oxygen tube in my nose, and a feeding tube. I was not prepared to hear the beeping of the cardiac and blood pressure monitors that continued to blare in my ear. As I took in the room more clearly, I saw pictures of my daughter, son-in-law, me with my five grandchildren, my husband,

and my dog. There were many questions pulsing through my brain: Why was I here? What happened? What day is it? What time is it? I saw a familiar face--that of my sister. I tried to cry out to speak but to my astonishment, had no voice but only a whisper. So I whispered, "I feel as though I just woke up from the dead." Her reply in a soft and gentle tone was, "Well, you kind of did." My sister explained that I had experienced a v-fib cardiac arrest and that I had been in the hospital for three and a half weeks. I simply could not hear anymore except to be sure my grandchildren had been taken care of by the Easter Bunny, which apparently I had missed. I realized my muscles had atrophied and I was so lethargic that is seemed impossible to get up, move, or do anything. Exhaustion took over from the news and weakness – so I went back to sleep in hopes of waking up after a terrible nightmare!

Looking back at that event, similar to what many of us have experienced, I have come to realize that in that restaurant was Michelle, an angel. Because of her medical training she was able to instruct my husband in artificial respiration, and perform CPR until the EMS unit arrived. The miracle of her being in the restaurant is the primary reason that I survived v-fib cardiac arrest, which claims 95% of its victims. When the EMS technicians arrived, they administered 2 shocks of the defibrillator and had me transported via U of M helicopter (Survival Flight) to the University of Michigan Hospital. They say that I received a $10,000 chopper ride, but was unconscious and unable to look out the window. I do believe them, as I received "wings" from the Survival Flight crew. (I think maybe U of M should offer patients who "missed out" on the experience of looking out the window, a free ride on their amazing helicopter. Seriously, what a thrill that would be!) ☺ All jokes aside, the extremely talented Survival Flight crew is incredible. They flew in the wind and bad weather to come to my rescue. I will always be in awe of their dedication and talent. As for Michelle, she is an angel, my guardian angel, and we are friends to this day. You see, there are wonderful people that will help you when there is a crisis situation and then continue in your life as your friend.

Upon arrival at U of M, I was quickly placed on the inner cool system (cooling of the blood) and a respirator as the wonderful doctors and staff used their skills and talents to revive me. Looking on with great care was my awesome Dr. Gregory Ensing, who kept my family informed of my progress and has always been there for me. I am certain it was a truly trying time for my family and friends. I always tell them that, "I wish I could have been there to help;" I guess I was! After 1 month, I was on my way home with an external defibrillator (a vest worn around the outside of the body), working to get strong for my upcoming heart surgery. Three months later, I had that surgery. Dr. Edward Bove and Dr. David Bradley were brilliant as they worked to insert a shunt (to help my original problem, pulmonary stenosis) and placed your friend and mine – the ICD. I have named my ICD – it is "Sparky."

Don't be afraid of your ICD. It is your friend and an insurance policy that we get to carry around inside our bodies. We are lucky to be able to say that! Having the device for almost 3 years- -even though I have not been shocked by the ICD (and pray I never am)-- doesn't necessarily come without incidents. I had recently purchased a "Smart Phone" from Verizon. It does everything: internet, movies, texting, and of course, phone calls. A few days after the purchase, I began hearing a chiming noise that seemed to follow me. This went on for 4 days until finally I decided to take the phone back to the store, figuring that something must have gone wrong with the battery. For a Smart Phone, you're pretty stupid, I kept thinking! Ironically, the same day I intended to return my phone, I received a call from the University of Michigan Hospital explaining that my defibrillator wires were having a problem! I thought, "What?! Are they kidding me?" As it turns out, I needed a thoracotomy to fix my fractured wiring! Ouch--a painful problem, but nothing I could not handle. Long story short – it was NOT my Smart Phone at all; it was my even smarter defibrillator trying to signal me that there was a problem. How amazing is that? In my life I've time-traveled from the "Dark Ages" of medicine, in which ether was a common anesthetic and we communicated using rotary dial telephones; to the era of today's modern technology in medicine, with sevoflurane as an anesthetic, and texting on Smart Phones!! Think of the possibilities for your future!

I also had an incident in a courthouse. I was there to support a friend during a traffic violation, and the officers would not frisk me, even though I had the appropriate paperwork. They insisted on using the magnetic scanner, which I refused. It was a bit of hassle but finally after a little complaining, I was allowed into the courthouse. Now the airport was a different matter – it was simply a BREEZE! I went through a scanner that uses radio waves and was in, out, and waiting for the rest of my family, less waiting for me! So, you see, there are some perks to being part of this "club" we belong to. ☺

Living with a defibrillator can sometimes be frightening and I will admit there have been times I've caught myself thinking, "Why me?" or that this just isn't fair. But then I stop and realize that life isn't always fair and I should count my blessings and continue living. That is the key – continue living. The ICD in my body is a life-saving device to help protect me against another cardiac arrest. I think of it as my friend, even though I am sometimes frightened. Most defibrillators are placed in the shoulder but "Sparky" is located in my abdomen. This is not the most flattering place for a woman to have a lump. But, I now can say that I have a good reason why I don't look as good in a bikini as I used to! ☺ Who knows, one day these ICDs may only be the size of a dime and then the lump in my abdomen may become fashionable. I could have a happy face painted on it, making it look like a tattoo or new piece of jewelry. More possibilities!

As positive as I sound, fear does exist. I am frightened daily concerning a shock from "Sparky" or that something else may go wrong. But I do not spend precious time worrying about what might be. I have already been there--to the point in life where things go very wrong--and I need and want to stay positive about where I am heading. So, I have been very active my entire life. I have always kept myself in good shape by working out, walking, riding horses, motorcycles, golfing, swimming, bowling, snorkeling, swimming with dolphins, and even parasailing. (Really I was not trying to give my cardiologist a heart attack.) But, you name it and I would try it-- within reason. Since my cardiac arrest and implantation of my ICD, I have needed to make modifications to tone down my activities. I still stay as active as possible, however, as I feel the importance of staying strong. I do count on my family and friends to support me. I must say I am extremely fortunate to have such wonderful medical care. My faith is strong and also has helped me through rough patches in my life, and to this day, I draw from the strength of faith and family to work, play and live.

People with "unique" hearts like ours are truly stronger than most. We are stronger emotionally, can be stronger physically, have a zest for life, and have more compassion and loving in our hearts because we understand what it is like to have physical limitations. I have been told by many that I am truly one of the strongest people they know, even among people with perfectly healthy hearts. I think this is true. We try harder, compensate for our physical limitations, and appreciate life more than the average bear! (I would much rather be a *unique* bear, than an *average* bear – wouldn't you?)

So, in closing, please be strong, live life to its fullest, stay positive, stay confident, and trust in your own strength. Moms and dads of heart patients: Allow your children to grow, encourage them to push themselves and stay as active as they can, and explain their limitations and conditions. Be patient with them. It will come back to you two-fold! Not only did I make it to adolescence, but I am living positively through adulthood. Children and teens: Push yourselves as much as you can (don't hurt yourself, of course), for as time goes on, you will be able to understand and realize your limitations. And young adults: By now, you know your limitations! There is much to be said for the "human spirit and will to live." Please don't be afraid to live your life! Embrace all the moments you possibly can from life; it is wonderful to be here. If I can do it without much correction of my heart, so can you! You have many more advantages and tons more technological assistance. I hope you can take some inspiration from my life to apply to your life.

I am honored to have the chance to reach out and I hope to touch at least one person. Giving you hope and encouragement, gives me hope and encouragement. Please never hesitate to reach out to me as I will be available to speak to you. I am proud to be a part of your life and am proud that you are reading about a small part of my life.

Let me leave you with this thought: In one of his songs, John Lennon wrote, *"Life is what happens to you while you are busy making other plans."* This is so true! So make your plans and don't be surprised if life happens somewhere in the middle! ☺

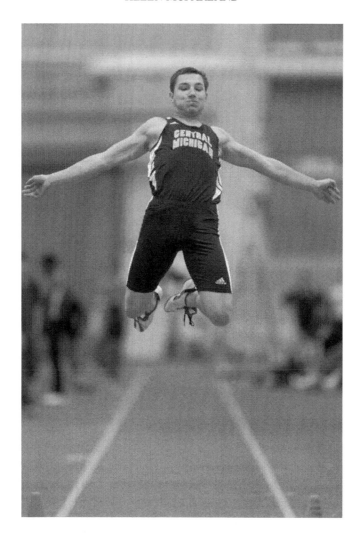

CHAPTER 7: FEARLESS

Brett

It was going to be the best weekend! There was anticipation for the "big game." Longtime rivals were going to bring together my family and friends to what has long been called "Central Western weekend." My parents had been planning the tailgate with friends and family. I was excited to have my best friend Chris come up from Western for the first visit of our freshman year in college. The early November football game was on a cold, fall Friday evening where some snow flurries were expected. You couldn't ask for a better setting for the big event.

I had a light track practice that day. We spent most of our time in the weight room lifting. After my mom set up at the tailgate, she and my sister Jenna walked over to the field house and watched me lift through the windows. As soon as I was finished with my workout, I walked over to the tailgate. I was a bit tired, having struggled with a cold for the past week or so. However, as soon as I had some food and saw my family and friends, I was energized for the night's events, at least that's what I thought. I had no idea that my life was about to take a major turn.

After tailgating for a few hours in the cold, we decided to forgo the game for the warmth of my dorm. We said our goodbyes to the families and my friends and I walked back to my dorm room to get warm. My mom remembers the last thing she saw was me riding piggyback on Chris's back, laughing and having a great time. Of course, as always, she said to us, "Make good choices!"

Back at my dorm room, as we were hanging out and just having some fun, Chris gets on my Facebook and writes "Brett loves Chris" on my status. I have learned about foreshadowing events in my English classes and if this isn't the best example of one, I'm not sure what is.

Soon after, we all headed to my friend Tyler's apartment. By now, it was about 9:30pm and the game was just about over. We watched the exciting finish on TV, as our parents were doing the same at the local pub. There is not much I remember from this point on in the story, and much of what preceded this has been retold to me so that I could remember. One minute I was standing at a table and the next I had fallen, face first onto the table, bruising my eye and landing unconscious on the floor.

As soon as I fell, Chris, not knowing what I was doing and thinking I was joking around like usual, turned me over. He saw my face was blue, realized I was gasping for breath and my eyes were rolled back, he yelled for someone to call 911. Tyler called right away. My friend Lauren began to cry and wasn't sure what to do. Chris knew right away that he needed to perform CPR. He began chest compressions and told Lauren to do the mouth to mouth breathing. Meanwhile, Tyler was on the phone with the EMS giving an account of my whereabouts, as well as my condition. Due to the fact that I was an 18 year old and it was one of the biggest college party nights of the year, it was assumed that I was having a reaction to drugs or alcohol. Little did anyone know at the time that I had had a sudden cardiac arrest.

Meanwhile, the police showed up after hearing the call. As soon as they saw me, they checked my pulse and did not feel one, so they told Chris that he could stop with the CPR. They told him that

I was dead. Chris got angry and said that he would not stop and continued with the CPR. This determination would eventually be what saved my life.

After about 15 minutes of CPR and talking with the EMS dispatch, the EMS arrived on the scene. They immediately took over and shocked me with the AED twice before taking me to the ER where my parents were waiting. Somehow in all the chaos, Chris had called my mom to tell her that I was on my way to the hospital. My parents arrived before me and were not able to see me right away as I needed to be shocked once again with the AED.

After doctors realized that I had a sudden cardiac arrest and needed to be at a hospital that was equipped to handle the trauma, they asked my parents if they wanted me transported to Grand Rapids or Saginaw. Thankfully, Chris's mom, who is a nurse, jumped right in with the decision to airlift me to the University of Michigan Hospital. As soon as I was on my way, my family left to make the trip themselves, not knowing what they would find upon arrival. Chris, Lauren and Chris's mom left for Ann Arbor as well.

Around 3:00am, I arrived in Ann Arbor where they immediately began the inter coolant system. I was brought to the CICU where I would lay in a coma for the next 58 hours. Through the grace of God and the excellent medical care from the U of M hospital staff, I survived my cardiac arrest. I awoke to a roomful of my family and closest friends. Confusion hit me; I didn't recognize anyone. Shortly, I began to regain my memory and a flood of over a hundred visitors came to see me. My Facebook page had blown up over the past few days and I had received more posts than someone would get on their birthday. Within the day, I regained controlled breathing on my own and was soon transferred to another area of the hospital.

Within the next couple of days, doctors would determine that I would need an ICD. On November 12, one week from the day I had my cardiac arrest, I would have the ICD implanted. There was no known cause of my cardiac arrest. An electrical issue with my heart was the best determination the doctors were able to make.

According to the rumors, it was from taking Adderall or it was from drinking Four Lokos. However, neither theory could be proven.

After my surgery, I was given one last night to stay in the hospital for recovery then was sent home. My best friends surprised me at my house. Still having no memory from the moment of my arrest, until after I got home, the next few days were spotty. I was told many stories of the hospital and still to this day hear stories of things I had done and do not remember. I was told that I was very humorous, which is a way to try and cope with what had happened. I tried to forget about the whole occurrence. However, the thought that I had cheated death made me feel supernatural. I went back to living life the way I had left it, with few minor changes.

Throughout the next 10 months, I lived life the way I would have before the arrest. A trip to Crystal Mountain with 16 of my closest friends was just what I needed to keep this off of my mind. Despite everyone's sympathy, I was able to put it behind me and live life without the effects of post-traumatic stress. With the 17 of us living so closely together, in a 2-bedroom, 6-person condo, time spent over the New Year was amazing. Snowboarding had been my favorite hobby since I learned how to ride when I was 9 years old.

After the winter break, I returned to Central Michigan to the start of my spring semester. I also got back to training with the track team with a couple of setbacks. I wasn't allowed to lift some parts of my upper body due to the implant of my ICD. However, I was back in the rhythm of long jumping, and had tied my personal best at the first indoor meet at 21' 9.5". Throughout the rest of the spring semester, I lived as though the cardiac arrest never happened.

Then summer came and I was back with my friends at home. Nothing makes me happier than to see them and we have a lot of fun together. Together, we don't make the best decisions but that's why I love them. Beach volleyball, swimming, bonfires, and longboarding take up most of our time. Unfortunately, on one of the first days of the summer, I had broken my wrist after a fall off my longboard. After being dragged by a car to have faster speed down a hill I got speed wobbles and jumped off. I was going about 35 mph, too fast to use my feet to run it off. I had to have three pins put in my wrist and had a cast on for 6 weeks. Once again, I didn't let this impact my life, so I went on having one of my favorite summers.

As August rolled in, everyone prepared to go back to school. I will always remember two days in my life. November 5, 2010 and August 15, 2011, the day I moved back to school. I woke up around 11am, packed up my Malibu, said goodbye to my family, and was off to Mt. Pleasant. After a near two-hour drive, I pulled into the city and turned toward my apartment. I noticed that my friend, Taylor, had an apartment in the complex right before mine. I stopped in to catch up with him; I hadn't seen him since May. Thirty minutes passed and I began to feel woozy. When I looked up, Taylor noticed it too. My face was pale. It was difficult to sit straight up. I thought it was nothing, so I played it off like I needed some fresh air. I asked Taylor to come longboard with me and we made our way out to the parking lot. But I still couldn't shake the feeling. I felt my heart beating out of my chest. I didn't know what to do, and paranoia set in. Taylor suggested that we head to the ER and within a minute, we were on our way.

The walk to the doors seemed like forever. With each step, it seemed like the doors were getting further away. After I checked in, I was seen immediately. A simple check of my pulse was all it took for the ER to swing into action. My standing heart rate was 164. I was put into a room and onto a bed. I was attached to one IV, then another, and then a third. There were several doctors rushing around me, talking fast. I felt like they were speaking another language, I couldn't understand them. But after a bag of fluids and an injection of some medicine that I still have no clue of the name, I was stable. Once again, the cause of this incident was unknown. An hour later I was released, it seemed like nothing big happened, so I wasn't worried. But I didn't know that this would affect who I was for the rest of the semester.

The day was over but not forgotten. The event was stuck in my head throughout the rest of the weekend. It was the worst thing that could've happened. The next weekend was supposed to be the most fun weekend of the summer. It was Welcome Weekend at

Central and since it was the first school to go back, friends from every school came to visit: Michigan, Michigan State, Western Michigan, Michigan Tech, and more. My three-bedroom apartment went from sleeping my two roommates and myself, to a group of near twenty. It was an amazing weekend, but the end of it wasn't expected at all. At around 5:30 on Sunday morning, we were just getting to sleep. However, I couldn't sleep. I was paranoid. I felt my pulse. Three rapid beats were followed by a pause, and then a couple, slower, beats. The irregular heartbeats are called tachycardia. I had my friends take me to the ER once again. Without hesitation, the doctors rushed to get me into a bed, but this time it was in the middle of a room where other patients could see. I was attached to a heart monitor, and again three IVs were put into my arms. Paranoia was getting the best of me.

Ten minutes passed and all I did was watch my heart monitor go from 60 to 90, back to 70, up to 95. Then a decision was made to have me airlifted to Saginaw. I let my parents know; at this point it was 6:15 in the morning. Not quite the wake-up call they were hoping for. I was exhausted myself; not having much sleep from the weekend of partying had drained me. I got on the helicopter and was so excited. It was my second time on a helicopter, but the first time I was able to remember it. At the time, I was stable, and just went through some tests when I arrived at Saginaw. I was released after a few hours, and was sent back to school.

For the next three months, I quickly went from a happy person to the lowest point I had ever been in my life. Depression quickly sunk in. I began to feel helpless. After the second week of class, I found myself sleeping in way past my classes. I easily spent over 14 hours a day in bed. I avoided contact with other people. I barely talked to anyone besides a few kids I knew from school. It affected my whole life. I began to have frequent flashbacks and had nightmares that would wake me up in the middle of the night with my heart pounding out of my chest. I was scared, frightened, and nervous to die. I thought I was going to die and I accepted that. I didn't care; I didn't try to reach out to anyone about it. My parents noticed that I wasn't doing too well in school, so they asked me why.

But I lied and said I was doing fine. Grades do not lie. They brought me home for the spring semester to try to get my head straight.

When I was home, my sister was the one who suggested that I try to take anti-depressants. I had been so miserable that I didn't even take advice from others, but for some reason, I listened to her. I went to the doctor and got a prescription for an anti-depressant pill. I took half a pill for the first five days, the doctor said the whole thing would be too much for me. He was right. After the third day, I felt happier. I was ready to take on the world. I was able to process thoughts in my head. I realized what I had to do with my life. It was as if this pill was the solution to all my problems. Throughout the next couple months, I continued to take the pills. It was an amazing change in direction for me. I started doing well in school. I read a book after my first class and wrote the book report that was due on the last day of class, over four months later. It was the first book I finished in over 10 years. I had never felt better in my life.

Don't take from this story that all you need is a pill to be better. It is not. I am currently not taking the pill because the things I have learned over the past few months of taking it have changed me. Don't live your life thinking negatively about your situation. Whether you had survived a cardiac arrest or have something wrong with your heart, you cannot let it affect who you are. Everybody loves to see you happy and they love to see you smile. Be productive. Don't be lazy. And certainly don't act like there is a time limit on your life. Get out and do something you have never done. Don't live in fear.

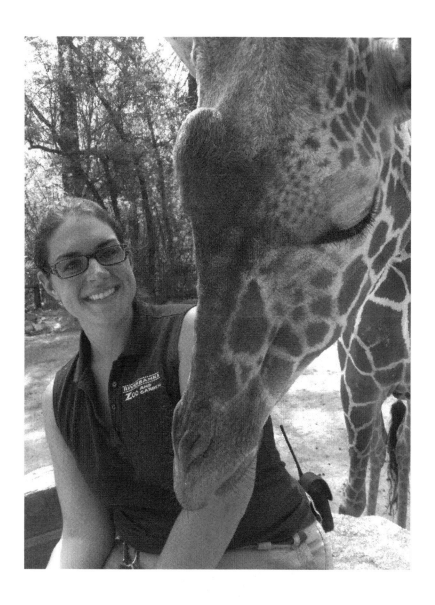

CHAPTER 8: MY JOURNEY WITH LQTS

Renee

I have always been a little different from your 'average' girl. Of course, I appreciate all things that glitter, and heaven help someone that messes up my hair, but I've always had an itch for adventure. So, when my 19th birthday rolled around, I wasn't about to hop the border to Canada like my other friends. Instead, I hopped on a train and headed west.

Philmont is a huge parcel of mountainous land in a remote area of New Mexico owned by the Boy Scouts of America. What many people don't know is that boy scouting is *not* just for boys. There is a branch of the BSA called Venturing, a coed youth-led group of which I was a part in 2007. My Venturing Crew had decided the year before that we wanted to conquer Philmont even though my intuition was telling me to stay home, this would not be an opportunity missed by any of us. After a 32-hour train ride, involving copious amounts of bad train food, card games, and some awkward sleeping positions, we made it to our destination.

On the morning of July 18, we gathered in the mess hall for our breakfast, took a group photo, and headed off for the trails. This was to be a weeklong trek of strenuous backpacking up and down mountains, over streams and rivers, and at the end of the day, into the comfort of our tents. The scenery was breathtaking and the trails, at points, seemed impossible. I joked to the group that if I made it home I would get a pint of Ben and Jerry's Chunky Monkey ice cream and watch the movie *Coyote Ugly*. I didn't realize that going home wasn't a guarantee.

After a few days, we made it to the peak of our first mountain. We took a group photo, sat and enjoyed the view before cooking up dinner. At this point, one of the cell phones had regained service and we all took turns and made a few calls. I called my mother to let her know where we were. I could tell she was worried. To be honest, I was too.

After supper we pitched our tents and hunkered down for the evening. It was the coldest night of the trip.

I woke up the next morning around 7am to the sound of my own voice. I wasn't talking in my sleep, I was screaming. I could hear myself howling and felt my body thrashing. I remember my inner monologue, "Why am I screaming? Just stop, STOP screaming. Just close your mouth. *Why can't I stop?*" Fear consumed me. I felt trapped in my own body. Then I heard the voice of one of the dads in the group. He was saying my name. I listened to him. I finally stopped screaming and lay still.

He was kneeling down beside me, looking scared. I noticed that my sleeping bag was wet. I had urinated on myself - needless to say this hadn't happened in many *many* years. No one knew what had happened. I had been screaming and thrashing for thirty minutes. I was embarrassed and terrified. I had no idea what had just happened or why.

One of the mothers said that her children had experienced night terrors and they looked something like what had just happened to me. The group decided that this was the best explanation. I knew it was unlikely for a 19 year old to suddenly develop night terrors, but we were at an un-staffed camp on the top of a mountain. There were no other options except to push on 10 miles to the next camp.

When we finally made it to the site I was relieved to see that it was a staffed camp. I could tell everyone else was relieved too. I washed my clothes and aired out my sleeping bag and took a much needed shower. We sat up until about 2am playing card games with our sister crew and then headed off to our tents. I remember waking up the next morning feeling warm and uncomfortable. I am thankful that I don't remember anything else.

According to my crew, around 5am it happened again—but much worse. They ran for help and I was taken by truck back to base camp to see a physician. By this point I was lucid and they asked me if I wanted to talk to my mom. I told them "no." I didn't want her to worry. The doctor told my mom that he thought I would be okay, but he wasn't sure what had happened. He was sending me to the hospital just in case. I was driven by ambulance to the closest hospital—about 80 miles away and as soon as I was admitted into the ER, I crashed. I was defibrillated and diagnosed with Long QT Syndrome (LQTS). This small hospital did not have the equipment to deal with this type of patient, so I was then taken by helicopter to the Heart Hospital of New Mexico in Albuquerque.

While I'm sure I enjoyed the drive and flight, I now try to vacation in slightly more populated areas.

From what I have been told, I was a bit of a difficult patient at the first hospital. Naturally, they pumped me full of drugs to calm me down. This was great for the doctors, but unfortunately the drugs masked my arrhythmia and the doctors at the Heart Hospital could not accept the diagnosis of LQTS since they couldn't see it for themselves. I was then put through what I like to call a real life episode of *House*. I was given multiple CTs, x-rays, blood tests, EKGs, and even a spinal tap. They just couldn't figure out what would make a 19-year-old woman go into ventricular fibrillation for no good reason. Luckily, when a nurse was changing my IV, I provided an answer for the doctors by coding once again. The prolonged interval shined bright as day on my monitor and was my ticket to my very own implantable cardioverter-defibrillator (ICD).

I now love and appreciate this little box that makes me feel just a little bit better than everyone else, but I haven't always felt this way. My implantation didn't exactly make me feel all warm and fuzzy inside.

Leaving the hospital I was very confused. The medications had severely impacted my short-term memory, and every time I looked down I needed to be reminded what happened, where I was, and why the pain was so excruciating. Remembering to take my pain-killers was the only thing that was not difficult.

The confusion lasted for about a week and I am thankful that everyone was so patient with me. The most difficult thing for me to deal with is the fact that there is a week of my life that I cannot remember to this day. Part of me wishes I knew what happened. Maybe I would have some clarity if I did, but the other part of me knows that if I truly had to live with those memories, I would be haunted by them. Instead, I enjoy the stories of mistaking my nurse for a "who" from the movie *The Grinch*. Like I said, they gave me *lots* of medication.

After returning home and once my short-term memory restored itself, I was back to the headstrong woman I had always been. Two weeks after I got my implant, I hopped on a train to Chicago to visit my cousin. This trip was planned before my adventure out west and there was no way I was going to let a "little" cardiac event stop me. I cannot believe my mother actually let me go after everything that had just happened, but I am so thankful she did. Immediately after returning from Chicago, I headed to East Lansing to begin my sophomore year at Michigan State University. I was determined not to let my fears of the unknown control me.

My ICD was just a speed bump, and If you've ever had the misfortune of driving with me, you know I don't slow down for those either.

Some speed bumps were larger than others. I remember the day that it all became real. It was the day I saw my scar. Because I had moved in early at MSU, there were only a few people in my dorm and, thankfully, I was alone in the community bathroom. I had finished my shower and as I toweled off I noticed that the sterile strips had finally loosened and were ready to come off. I stood in front of the mirror. I just stood there. Staring at the loosened strips, terrified to see what lay beneath. I finally worked up the courage to peel them off.

I cried. I stood in front of the mirror and cried. I must have been hoping that there wouldn't be a noticeable scar. Or that maybe the whole thing had been put in through one *very* small pin-hole. Obviously this was not the case.

I now know that my scar looks similar to everyone else's. It is above my left breast, and is about an inch and a half long. I hated it at the time, but I now just accept it as a part of me, just like a mole or a birthmark. And I decided that I would not hide my scar (mostly because this would involve an entirely new wardrobe) and that I would do my best to embrace it. Everyone has battle wounds; ICD patients are the lucky ones who get to show them off every day.

Living with an ICD changes things. Feeling like I lost control over my life was my greatest struggle. Between doctor's visits, random excruciating pain, and the constant fear that I might get shocked, I felt helpless. I had to learn to work through it.

According to state law, I was not allowed to operate a vehicle for six months. To me, this was worse than hearing the news that I nearly died twice. Six months. No driving. It seems silly looking back, but I was heartbroken at the time. A vehicle was freedom. The simple fact that I *could not* drive completely overruled the fact that I didn't really need to. I was in school, there was adequate public transportation, and, if I ever needed to go home for the weekend, my mother was more than happy to pick me up. Sometimes logic escapes an ailing mind.

Living in fear also made me feel like my life was no longer in my own control. I am fortunate enough that I have not had any episodes since my initial cardiac arrests, and I have also not experienced any inappropriate shocks. The most difficult fear to overcome was the device itself. I have no reason to doubt my ICD, but the possibility that it could send 32 Joules through my body at any given moment can be a little nerve wracking.

One of the first weekends back at Michigan State I spent the night on the futon in the room of my two best friends, Mark and

Sam. We had previously gone to an orientation event called "Sparticipation" where we collected copious amounts of junk from various student organizations. Most of this junk consisted of organization flyers, chip clips, pens, and the dreaded refrigerator magnet. I know that a magnet must be pretty large to affect an ICD, but 4-weeks-post-surgery Renee did not fully trust that. I had made sure that all refrigerator magnets were in a bag on the opposite side of the room before I went to bed, but I woke up in the middle of the night and decided that this was not good enough because I had forgotten the ones actually stuck to the refrigerator. I made quite a fuss until both Sam and Mark were both trying to calm me down and remind me that I was going to be just fine. I have since realized that most of my fears regarding my ICD were unwarranted. It is there to keep me safe, and so far it has done exactly that.

After about nine months I was much more comfortable with my ICD. I had accepted my new restrictions and was ready for a new adventure. Less than a year after my implant, I took off to Tampa, Florida, for a four month internship at Busch Gardens.

My implant site was still healing and the drastic change in weather seemed to upset the area a little. I quickly found a heart clinic in the area and went for a checkup. The clinic waiting room was something I had become accustomed to. The ladies at the desk always comment on my age and tell me I'm "too young to have heart problems." Then I take a seat in a room full of people my grandmother's age. I finally saw the doctor and he told me I had "healing pains." Take my word for it: these pains felt remarkably unhealthy. I had experienced pains like this right after my implant and I actually left a Detroit Tigers baseball game and ran out of Comerica Park when the pains hit. I felt like I was dying. No one ever told me that the pain would last for a year and a half, but trust me, it can.

I am now approaching my fifth year with my ICD. I finished a B.S. in Zoology at Michigan State University and was hired shortly after graduation into my dream job working at a zoo with babirusa, elephants, giraffes, kangaroo, ostrich, wallaby, vultures, and zebra. I know it's that little box of technology that made it possible. And I am grateful, even though it can be a bit of a burden at times.

The doctor I saw in Florida said something to me that changed my life. He asked to shake my hand and said, "You are a survivor and I am grateful for meeting you." I had never thought of myself in that way, but he was right. We are all survivors, emergency implant or not. We have defied nature and pulled through life-threatening conditions.

I have learned that every challenge the ICD has and will present, is *much* better than the alternative.

Keep on beating.

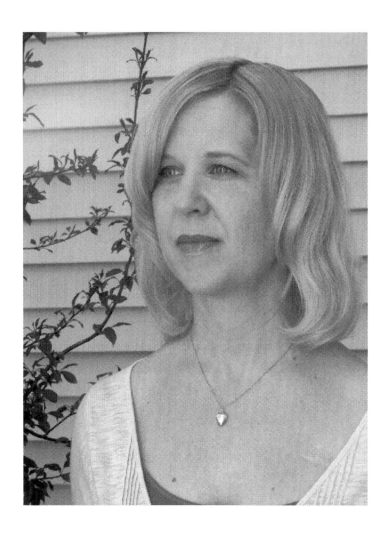

CHAPTER 9: MY RHYTHM OF LIFE
Lisa

"Hmmmm…" That's never a comforting sound from a physician. But, that was exactly what my primary care doctor said as she looked over the ECG tape from the test she had just administered.

I had gone in for a yearly physical with a new doctor whom I hadn't been to before. After listening to my heart, she asked if I was a long-distance runner or if I had ever been told I had a murmur. When I answered no to both, she thought it would be a good idea to have an ECG, which I never had before. After looking at the tape, she told me she wanted me to see a cardiologist right away and made an appointment for me.

At only 21 years old, I was trying not to worry but was actually freaking out inside. I had a normal childhood, played sports and never had any kind of medical problem other than chicken pox and the flu. A cardiologist? Right away? I figured there was no way this was a good thing.

After seeing the cardiologist and having stress tests, echocardiograms and other tests, the cardiologist informed me that I had third-degree, or complete, congenital heart block. In layman's terms, the top and bottom chambers of my heart had no electrical conduction to cause them to beat with each other and instead were beating independently. Although I never had symptoms, it was something I was born with. I was stunned. How could no one have ever diagnosed this? How could I never have known? What did it mean? Was I going to die? Quite frankly, I was terrified.

The doctor explained that it was a very rare condition that was often fatal in newborns. At the time, (the late 1980s) he said he couldn't explain why some people, myself included, didn't have severe symptoms and had hearts that compensated for the electrical malfunction. He suggested the best course of action was to have yearly checks wearing a 24-hour monitor and alert him immediately if I developed any symptoms like lightheadedness, inability to exert myself or passing out. He then explained that at some point in my life I would probably become symptomatic and need a pacemaker.

What? Aren't pacemakers for old people? And would I have to give away my microwave? That was pretty much all I knew about pacemakers. After my initial shock and fear, I did what he said and just went on with my life, rarely thinking about this strange disorder I had.

Fast forward almost 20 years. I still hadn't developed any symptoms. In fact, I had gotten somewhat lax in being timely with yearly checks. I had moved, switched doctors and nothing changed. Doctors still couldn't understand why I worked given my condition. No matter the doctor, I was always the only patient they had with my disorder.

Then one day my mom asked me when I had last seen a cardiologist. I realized it had been more than a year. I also realized that strangely enough, I had never searched the Internet on my condition. When I did, I found a recent academic paper about my condition exactly. Reading the words, "In many asymptomatic cases, the first symptom is sudden cardiac death," was not exactly the comfort I was looking for. In fact, all the worries I had from that first diagnosis came rushing back at full speed. I contacted the researcher and surprisingly, he wrote back immediately and urged me to see an electrophysiologist and suggested the University of Michigan Health System would be an excellent place to go.

I was pretty scared but once I met my doctor, Eric Good, I immediately relaxed. First of all, he was very knowledgeable about my condition and had treated many other patients with the same thing. It felt so much better to know there were others such as me who had been successfully treated by this doctor. He recommended a pacemaker to create the electrical pulses that my heart could not do properly on its own. Given that I was really not interested in exploring the sudden cardiac death "symptom," I scheduled the surgery.

I realized then how important it was to have a doctor whom I trusted completely and who listened intently to my concerns and wishes. He explained everything in terms I could understand, assured me that my worries about how the device would look were normal and OK and that he would do his best to hide my device. Most of all, he made me feel like a partner and not just a patient.

I had my pacemaker implanted a week after I turned 40. Getting a pacemaker for your 40th birthday isn't the best way to celebrate, but I realized I was lucky to be able to celebrate at all given the chances I had taken with my heart for all those years. In the back of my mind, I had always known this was a possibility, so emotionally I managed pretty well. My doctor kept his word and did an outstanding job of making the device hardly noticeable. I recovered quickly and started to adjust to living with a device.

Things seemed to be going well when I had a checkup five months later. I visited the office and Laura, a wonderful device clinic nurse, ran through the tests. Though she didn't say, "Hmmmm," while looking at the report, I could tell something wasn't right. She left and later came back with a doctor whom I didn't know. Dr. Good wasn't in the office that day but there was a concern with my results. It seemed that the pacemaker had actually recorded an additional problem with my heart while I was sleeping – an episode of ventricular tachycardia – that was very dangerous and could result in sudden cardiac death. I was told it was something that couldn't be controlled with the pacer alone and that I would need to either have cardiac ablation or have my pacer replaced with an Implantable Cardioversion Defibrillator.

I was completely thrown for a loop. In my mind, I had finally gotten my pacer and taken care of my problem. How could I possibly have another problem that put me at high risk? Wasn't one enough? It was all extremely overwhelming and I was terrified that the V-tach would happen again before they had a chance to try ablation. It didn't help that my doctor wasn't there to deliver the news, but it did help to have Laura there. I remember her asking if I needed her to drive me home — probably forgetting that I live an hour from the hospital. I made it home by myself that day, amid a snow storm and a lot of crying.

Dr. Good contacted me within a few days and arranged for me to be fitted with a Life Vest, an external defibrillator that is worn strapped to the body at all times. Needless to say, it was quite the fashion statement when worn with lovely holiday dresses that season. Then again, it was there to save my life and made the wait before my procedure much less stressful.

I went in to the hospital about six months after receiving my pacemaker so that my doctor could try cardiac ablation to take care of the area that was causing my V-tach. I knew going in that if he wasn't successful with it, my pacer would have to be replaced with an ICD. I was terrified of the very idea of having an ICD and had convinced myself I wouldn't need it. I knew that they were bigger, had a shorter battery life, and — oh yeah — could administer a huge shock to my body that had been compared to being kicked by a horse. In my head, I knew that I would get what I needed to keep me safe but my emotions kept telling me that I didn't want any of this. I simply wanted to go back to a time when I thought I was "normal" and not a "heart patient."

I woke up from surgery and immediately put my hand to the left side of my chest. Yep...there was the same bulky bandaging I had had just six months earlier. I knew then that the ablation hadn't worked and I was now the new recipient of something I didn't want — an ICD. Because the drugged haze I was in, I don't remember much more from the recovery room but I was told later (by the psychologist consult that showed up at my bedside) that I was pretty angry and yelling about how I didn't want an ICD. Awesome. Not only did I have to get an ICD but I embarrassed myself by yelling so much they assumed I needed a psychologist.

Since I had just been through the same recovery six months earlier, I knew exactly what to expect and prepared accordingly. I remembered a strapless bra, I took my meds before the pain started, I wore clothes that were easy to get into and I had prepared things at home so I wouldn't have any reaching to do. The one thing I wasn't prepared for was my emotional state. This time my emotions were so different, but I couldn't really figure out why. I couldn't stop crying. I couldn't stop thinking about the device in my chest. And then I got angry with myself for crying and not being strong enough to soldier on like nothing had happened. I didn't understand why I managed with the pacemaker so well and this was bothering me so much.

Again, Dr. Good had been absolutely wonderful. My incision was minimal and he managed to hide my device so that there was no discernible lump that I had been worried about. He visited my room the day after my surgery and said all the right things. Physically, everything was wonderful and recovery was relatively easy. (Well, except for that maize and blue University of Michigan sling they sent me home with to East Lansing. This lifelong Spartan had a lot of explaining to do. It's my heart, not football, so yes, I went to U-M).

And yet still, something wasn't right with me. I tried talking with family and friends. They tried to be supportive and understanding, but still no one really understood what I was going through. Thinking they were being helpful, some told me I was lucky and that I should just get on with my life. In my head I knew that was true, but I really didn't feel all that lucky at the time.

To this day I still can't really put my finger on why I was so sad and worried for months after my surgery. I know now that there was nothing to blame, nothing I did wrong. Emotional rollercoasters are a very normal part of any health challenge, and every patient has the right to feel however he or she feels and work through those emotions in whatever way he or she needs to. No one is the same, and no one deals with anything exactly the same. And no one should ever tell someone, "Just forget about it." When you're the patient, doing so is much easier said than done.

Dr. Good was extremely compassionate and understanding. He knew that my whole self, not just my heart, needed care and suggested I go to a counselor.

Through my employee assistance program at Michigan State University, I was able to see a wonderful counselor. He let me talk. He let me cry. He told me my feelings were valid. He gave me coping skills. He helped me work out why I was so angry and sad. He gave me ways to talk with family and friends to express what I needed from them. He made me feel like I was entirely normal. And, most importantly, on the day of my last session, he told me he was proud of me. That was the day I realized I was proud of myself and that I had been given a great chance at a wonderful life.

I've had my ICD for five years now, and I've never been shocked. I'm still paced almost 100% of the time. Do I still have moments or days when I worry? Absolutely. Who wouldn't in my situation? But, it's just a new part of what makes me, me. I'm not shy about it. I use my situation to educate people. I used to hide my scar. Now I wear it proudly. I've participated in conferences to meet others with ICDs and have met some amazing women who have become great friends. I've spoken at employee training sessions at the UMHS. I've joined a patient family-centered care advisory council to help improve patient experiences even more.

I enjoy my family and friends. I work hard. I play hard. I don't let my condition or my device slow me down.

I remember when I was asking Dr. Good about the limitations I might have with my ICD. After talking about standard things like MRIs, magnets, etc., he told me something I try to remember every day. "I put your ICD in you so you could live. So go do that. Live."

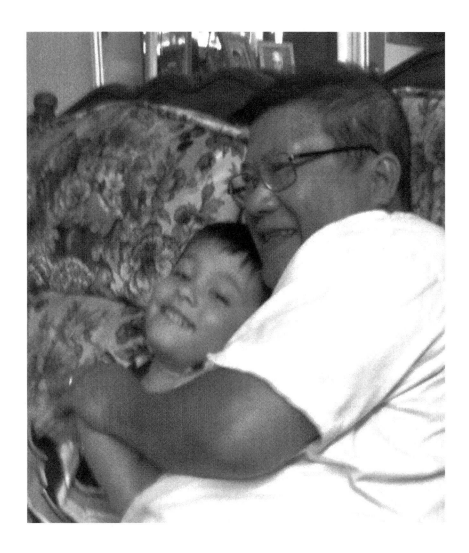

CHAPTER 10: BY THE NUMBERS
Michelle

Family Summer Vacation August 2008 Pentwater, Michigan: Our extended family had been vacationing for a week in a cottage at Pentwater, Michigan. It had been almost a decade since our entire family, (my husband and son, joined by both my parents, and 2 sisters with their husbands), have taken an entire week vacation trip. It was picture perfect. The weather was nice each day we walked down to the sandy shore. My mom, who brought along her pots and pans to this rental cottage, along with her Filipino spices and magical mystery ingredients, would wake us up to traditional breakfasts, and serve us delectable lunches and dinners for the entire week. My dad brought along his fishing poles, binoculars, goggles & flippers, to enjoy the sandy beaches of Lake Michigan.

My parents, Alvaro (then 65) and Christina (then 60), born and raised in the Philippines, immigrated here in the United States in 1992. They were raised from a time and culture that didn't complain much, and was happy and content with the simple joys in life. They brush off little aches and pains here and there, thinking that it comes with age, and that it will somehow go away with rest and sleep.

On one of the afternoons during this vacation, we all took a stroll down to the beach. There was a lighthouse at the end. We also found a trail that turns into flights of wooden steps that leads up to a high perch overlooking Lake Michigan with its gorgeous sunset viewing area.

As we headed down the trail, my dad paused midway through the flat sandy path, and told us he felt "too tired" and wouldn't be able to catch up with us on this activity. He told us he just wanted to relax, wanted for us to go on. We have all been pretty active throughout this vacation, exploring the town and walking down to the beach every day. So, we really didn't think too much of this hesitation on his part. But my husband and I (both nurses at U of M), did take a little pause at that fact, and stored that mental image in the back of minds. I say this, because this will eventually play a role in putting pieces of the puzzle that will unfold later. Even to this day, that moment rings clear in our memory.

Christmas season came. At the end of our family dinner, my dad sat on the couch and started tapping his arms. I took notice and asked him why he was doing that. He said both arms just feel tired and a little numb. My mom said she also saw my dad looked like he was short of breath just with getting ready to go out and putting on his coat and stuff. That then cued me to know that something was wrong. I called for the next available clinic appointment to get him seen by his doctor.

I accompanied him to his primary doctor to get him checked. In the exam room, I related to his doctor, the signs and symptoms I had noticed, even recalling his comment of "feeling tired" from walking on the sandy beach of Pentwater, Michigan. His doctor orders an EKG to be done right then and there. Needless to say, after he saw the print out from the machine, we didn't end up going home that day, but instead going to the emergency room. He was then admitted to the University of Michigan ER, where he was ordered for a stat Echocardiogram at the bedside.

Here were his revealing results from that study:

Echo Report Case Date: 10/24/2008 Report Date: 10/24/2008 University of Michigan Health System / Cardiovascular Center Adult Echocardiography Laboratory

Portable Transthoracic Echo -- Acquired
Referring Location: Emergency Department
Indications: Chest Pain, Unspecified (2D, SE), Abnormal EKG (2D, SE)
PROCEDURE INFORMATION
Performing Location: Emergency Department
Sonographer _____
Priority: Stat   Status: Emergency Department
Modalities:
-- Color Doppler
-- Spectral Doppler MEASUREMENTS
LVIDd: 60 mm LVIDs: 55 mm
IVSd: 12 mm   LVPWd: 12 mm
LA: 38 mm
LV EF: 20/ Estimated

VALVES
AORTIC VALVE
Anatomy: Focally thickened, without stenosis
Regurgitation: Minimal
MITRAL VALVE
Anatomy: Restricted mitral valve leaflets.
Regurgitation: Mild to moderate
TRICUSPID VALVE
Anatomy: Anatomically normal
Regurgitation: Minimal, may be within normal limits Estimated RV Systolic
pressure of 36 mmHg based on estimated RA pressure of 5 mmHg.
PULMONIC VALVE
Anatomy: Grossly normal
Regurgitation:

CHAMBERS AND FUNCTION NOTES:
Left ventricular hypertrophy.
Left ventricular enlargement
Abnormal septal motion consistent with post--operative state and bundle branch
block.
Severely decreased left ventricular systolic function. Normal overall right
ventricular systolic function. Inferior wall akinetic.

AORTA
Grossly normal as seen

PERICARDIUM
Pericardial Effusion: None

CONCLUSIONS
Severely decreased left ventricular systolic function
(Full--thickness myocardium)

Mild--to--moderate mitral regurgitation.

Needless to say, after seeing all these, and consulting with the doctor in the ER, it looked pretty shocking and grim. My dad went from being able to witness the birth of his first grandchild (Lance, then 4 years old), and looking forward to years of sharing Lance's childhood and more with him, to maybe looking at shortening that span to about a year. My husband, who also worked as a nurse in the electrophysiology lab back then, painted a grim but realistic future to our family members.

Looking at the labs and test results, it didn't bode well for my dad. I understood what the numbers meant and could translate them to the saddening fact that we may not have my dad for long in our lives. He is now looking at heart failure with an ejection fraction of 20.

Looking back in August of 2008 at our Pentwater family vacation and fast forward that to 4 months, and having the following findings...
-coronary heart disease
 -dilated cardiomyopathy
-severely depressed left ventricular systolic function
-estimated ejection fraction of 20-25%
-New York Heart Association class 2-3 Heart Failure symptoms

The one blessing about this was being at the University of Michigan Hospital, Cardiovascular Center. It is a facility that has all the resources you could think of, and all are there available to you as a patient and as a family member. The staff is all knowledgeable and well versed in their fields of expertise. My dad's admission in the emergency room, and the number of cardiac diagnoses he obtained triggered the systematic array of collaboration that was immediately set up, as part of being under the system of health care management at U of M. There would be the integration and coordination between his primary doctor (with Dr. McMaster), the electrophysiology department (with Dr. Good), and the introduction and management of the Heart Failure Clinic (with Dr. Koelling), to comprise his entire cardiac care team. My dad and mom would also eventually develop a good relationship as well, with the device nurses and staff at the clinic for his follow up and checks. This was such a tremendous benefit being at this facility. The communication, expert skills, and dedication from each of these services were outstanding.

Part of my dad's cardiac care involved being placed and managed by the heart failure clinic. He was put on a number of medications, each controlled and monitored by their skilled staff. Each and every medication was explained as far as what they do, and what lab values they can look at that would let them know how effective it was working and helping his heart function.

I could remember my dad noting one of the medication he identifies as the pill that "helps his heart muscle get that extra squeeze" at end of every pulse. Things the staff help explain it like that, help the non-medical person understand what the meds they are taking and why.

For the scientifically minded reader out there, this type of medical management aided in providing an outstanding improvement of my dad's heart failure status. One evidence is from his BNP results, which the heart failure clinic monitored every time. Keep in mind his starting BNP on admission was 368. I will reveal his latest numbers towards the end, along with the other empirical data.

B-type natriuretic peptide (BNP) is a cardiac neurohormone secreted from membrane granules in the cardiac ventricles as a response to ventricular volume expansion and pressure overload.

Levels of atrial natriuretic peptide (ANP) and BNP are elevated in cardiac disease states associated with increased ventricular stretch. Levels above 200 pg/ml, however, would almost always indicate left heart failure.

March 2009, University of Michigan Cardiovascular Center: Under the skilled and expert care of Dr. Good, my dad would receive a Dual Chamber Biventricular ICD.

A special kind of pacemaker, called a biventricular pacemaker, is designed to treat the delay in heart ventricle contractions. It keeps the right and left ventricles pumping together by sending small electrical impulses through the leads. This therapy, also called resynchronization therapy, has been shown to improve the symptoms of heart failure and the person's overall quality of life. Re synchronization therapy is one part of a comprehensive heart failure management program. Medications, diet, lifestyle change, and close follow-up with a heart failure specialist, combined with device and/or surgical therapy, will help reduce symptoms and allow the patient to live a more active life.

During the time of my dad's implantation procedure, while waiting, my mom and I took a stroll through the small library that was on the 1st floor of the Cardiovascular Center (CVC). It's called "the Friends with a heart gift shop." We found so much materials and resources, that were available to the patients and their families, all jam packed into such a small space. They even had models and pictures of the heart and its anatomy, and samples of different pacemakers and defibrillators for the public to view and touch. Books lined the shelves. Pamphlets abound the walls for all the different heart problems and all other information one might need to avail of. I could even remember the volunteer worker in that shop asking me that time, if I needed anything, and that if I couldn't find a book or material I wanted, she could obtain and borrow it from the other university libraries around the campus. I thought to myself, even I, a nurse who had worked there for more than a decade and a half, am truly impressed being on the receiving end of the care we strive to always provide to our patients.

My dad's procedure and recovery went well. With the system in place at the CVC, follow ups and everything were set up for him at discharge. It included clinic appointments with the heart failure department, his primary physician, and now, with the Device clinic.

A few weeks after my dad's procedure, I could tell by his non-verbal cues, that he was still adjusting to having the bi-V ICD implant. It felt to him as if something "foreign" was now residing inside his body. His device was also implanted sub- muscularly, meaning, it stuck out a bit from his upper chest. We could see slightly, the edges of the little "generator outline" protruding under his skin. For my dad, it wasn't only knowing the fact that a "foreign body" was inside of him now, but he could also see it in the mirror, and feel it with his hand. For quite a while, I could see him massage his upper left chest where the device generator was. Maybe it was to coax it and have it in his mind, that "it" was now part of him. This adjustment did take a while to overcome. What helped him tremendously was knowing that he was not alone in this venture.

With the system in place at the Cardiovascular Center, they are not only concerned with the surgical and medical part of the diagnoses and schematics. They are also concerned with the psychological aspect and the impact of having a cardiac device implanted. Within their device clinic, they have built and structured a number of organized support systems. They introduced not only my dad, but my mom and the entire family, to the ICD support group.

My mom and dad attend these sessions held throughout the year. The Device clinic pools in resources, invites knowledgeable speakers, and collaborates with other patients and their family members to join, comfort, and encourage one another, as they go through living life with an implantable device. Then there's the big annual June Device picnic that my parents always look forward to. My mom always makes sure she has that day off. My dad and mom are able to talk to other patients/families who share the same path. That is how much they look forward to these events. Believe me when I say, it DOES really help, to know you have support out there. I know it has helped my parents. The clinic also has a support group that targets young patients who have received their device at an early age. I have been invited to volunteer along with my husband at one of the events they sponsor for the kids. They call this annual event "Young ICD Connection." Being around these kids, I witnessed how they all develop a sense of comradeship with each other, and the way the entire device clinic provides support to their families. It really proved and showed their commitment to their "device support program, kids and grown-ups alike."

I would like to start closing this chapter with the Ex post facto test results revealing how well my dad recovered and benefited from being under the care of the heart failure clinic and the Device clinic. The Bi-Ventricular device, coupled with the excellent care he obtained from the heart failure clinic, have returned years of life that my dad would've lost, knowing the condition we were presented with in the Emergency room. We were staring at heart failure and a complete halt of his golden years, to being given back time and years with his grandson Lance.

As of now, my dad is only seen at the heart failure clinic once a year, since his heart has responded remarkably and recovered well. I remember about 2 years ago, Dr. Koelling saying to my dad at the last visit I accompanied him with, "well looking at your numbers, I only need to see you once a year now..."

By the way, his BNP lab result from"368" at the emergency room admission in 2008, to now "15" at best !!! (Can we get a "whoa" here?)

Here are his post Device Echo studies/results:

Other Results Text --? Test Name: Echo Report Case Date: 11/17/2009 Report Date: 11/19/2009 University of Michigan Health System / Cardiovascular Center Adult Echocardiography Laboratory
TTE -- Acquired
Referring Location: 150 -- Cardiovascular Medicine
Indications: Cardiomyopathy (2D, SE, TEE)
PROCEDURE INFORMATION
Performing Location: Canton Health Center
Priority: RoutineStatus: Outpatient
 Equipment: Acuson Sequoia Modalities:
-- Color Doppler
-- Spectral Doppler
Quality of Study: Adequate

MEASUREMENTS
LVIDd: 46 mm LVIDs: 25 mm
IVSd: 12 mm   LVPWd: 13 mm
LA: 35 mm   LA area: 13.4 cm2
LV EF: 65 / Estimated (here lies the proof in the pudding !!!)
AORTA
Annulus: Sinus: 31 mm SinoTubular:

Tubular: Arch:
VALVES
AORTIC VALVE
Anatomy: Thickened aortic valve without stenosis
Regurgitation: No evidence of aortic regurgitation Peak gradient: 6 mmHg
MITRAL VALVE
Anatomy: Calcified mitral annulus
Regurgitation: Minimal, may be within normal limits E/A ratio: 0.7
Decel time: 143 msec

TRICUSPID VALVE
Anatomy: Anatomically normal
Regurgitation: Mild
Estimated RV Systolic pressure of 34 mmHg based on estimated RA pressure of 5 mmHg.
PULMONIC VALVE
Anatomy: Grossly normal
Regurgitation: No evidence of pulmonic insufficiency
CHAMBERS AND FUNCTION
Left Atrium: Normal Size Right Atrium: Normal Size
Left Ventricle: Normal Size
LV Hypertrophy: Mild, concentric
Right Ventricle: Normal Size
NOTES:
Normal overall left ventricular systolic function. Normal overall right ventricular systolic function. Normal wall motion.

AORTA
Anatomically normal
PERICARDIUM
Pericardial Effusion: None
MISCELLANEOUS
Pacemaker lead in the right atrium and right ventricle.
CONCLUSIONS
Normal left ventricular systolic function.

Interpreted Date: 11/17/2009

My dad, our entire family, and especially his grandson Lance, would like to express our appreciation for the excellent care the University of Michigan Cardiovascular Center has provided. I being an empirical person, the year 2008 had my dad staring at the reality and repercussions of having an ejection fraction of 20-25 %, and heart failure. Now, he is thriving with a staggering EF of 65 % and THAT translates to years given back, to be spent fishing, vacationing, and playing chess with his grandson, Lance.

Frequently Asked Questions about Implantable Cardioverter Defibrillators (ICDs)

Laura Horwood, NP
University of Michigan Hospital

Q. What is an implantable cardioverter defibrillator?
An implantable cardioverter defibrillator (ICD) is an implantable device that provides immediate therapy to a life-threatening arrhythmia (heart beating too quickly) via a sequence of painless impulses or a jolt of electricity. It can also act as a pacemaker if the heart is beating too slowly.

Q. Why might a person need one?
Numerous underlying heart conditions that can cause a weakening of the heart muscle can predispose an individual to develop or be at risk to develop life threatening ventricular arrhythmias. For adults, the most common condition is coronary artery disease leading to ischemic cardiomyopathy (where the heart can't pump enough blood to the rest of the body). There are also a number of inherited conditions that can cause a person to have sudden life threatening ventricular arrhythmias. Examples include: Hypertrophic Cardiomyopathy, Long QT Syndrome, Brugada Syndrome, and Arrhythmogenic Right Ventricular Cardiomyopathy.

Q. How does it work?

The implantable device continuously monitors the heart's rhythm and is programmed to deliver "pacing impulses" to restore its natural rhythm, which would avoid the need for a shock. If pacing is unsuccessful, it will deliver a shock to the heart.

Q. Where does it get implanted?

The device is implanted under the superficial skin tissues in a preformed pocket in the left or right chest area (just under the collar bone). The leads are inserted into the large subclavian vein and threaded into the heart and then secured within the right heart chambers.

Q. How does my doctor determine if I need an ICD?

Through a comprehensive evaluation that includes: history and physical exam, echocardiography (using sound waves to see the heart), and electrocardiography (measures heart's electrical impulses). Sometimes the individual may require further tests such as a nuclear stress test, cardiac catheterization and cardiac MRI.

Q. How big is it?

It's slightly smaller and thinner than a pager.

Q. How much is the ICD going to protrude from my chest?

It depends on the person. It also depends on the type of implant that you receive. Some of the implants are very small and some are a little bigger. If you're thin, it generally will protrude. If you have a little more bulk it won't be so obvious. The device can be implanted under the chest muscle, which would prevent it from being seen. Speak to your physician about options for your implant location.

Q. What does a shock feel like?

Some people say they felt like they were kicked in the chest by a horse. Others describe the shock as it feels like being hit in the back with a hard object. Still others say it wasn't as bad as they expected. In general, patients will agree that the shock is uncomfortable, however, it is quick and there is no lingering discomfort.

Q. What should I do after a shock?

First thing, you should sit down. It's possible that you could pass out from the arrhythmia, and you want to make sure you don't fall and/or hit your head. Call your doctor's office and let them know you received a shock. When patients know they received a therapy (pacing or shock), it is important to have the device evaluated to make sure the device is working properly and to document your arrhythmia episode. Your device may be evaluated remotely by a home monitor. However, if you have received multiple shocks or you are having symptoms, you will be directed to your doctor's office or the emergency room to be evaluated.

Q. Can I still work with an ICD?

That depends on what you do for a living. Most people with an ICD are able to continue working. Speak with your doctor about your occupation.

Q. Will people be afraid to touch me?

No. Even if someone does touch you when you are shocked, it won't hurt the other person. They may feel a tingle, like getting a static shock.

Q. I feel scared and depressed. Is this normal?

This is absolutely normal. In the beginning, many people worry about having arrhythmias and if and when a shock will happen. You have also been diagnosed with a new medical condition and have undergone a surgical procedure. This new diagnosis will also likely impact many areas of your life. This is a major event in your life and many individuals go through an adjustment period. Joining a support group and meeting others who share your fears can be beneficial. If you're experiencing anxiety, you can speak to your doctor about anti-anxiety medication and/or counseling to help you through this transitional period.

Psychosocial Factors Related to Living with an Implantable Cardioverter Defibrillator and Proposed Strategies for Success

Lauren D. Vazquez, PhD

Coping with treatment with an implantable cardioverter defibrillator (ICD) can certainly be considered a life-changing experience. As with any significant life event, the process of adjustment can be challenging. Research has shown that ICD patients face common difficulties after implantation of their device. My work as a clinical health psychologist has been focused on identifying those difficulties and helping patients develop strategies to adjust to treatment adaptively and embrace the best quality of life possible. The purpose of this chapter is to describe the psychosocial concerns that are common in ICD patients and to propose a set of coping skills that can help you be more successful in living life to the best of your ability.

Psychosocial Concerns

Life may bring many stresses over time as we experience change, loss, or hardship. Coping with treatment with an ICD may represent one of those changes that you find stressful. Stress is a term to describe the entire set of challenges, frustrations, and changes that we all deal with on a daily basis. We know that ICD patients cope with a unique set of stressors that may create an equally unique set of concerns. Approximately 15% of patients will experience what is considered significant emotional distress (Sears et al., 1999). Distress may include anxiety (often centered on the potential for ICD shock), depression, family concerns, or other device-specific adjustment difficulties. Risk factors for distress include being female, being young (under the age of 50), patients with limited social support, those with a limited understanding of their heart condition or how their ICD functions and those patients who have a previous history of ICD shock (Sears & Conti, 2002). However, while psychological distress may not be uncommon, research suggests that overall ICD patients generally report good quality of life (Schron et al., 2002; Irvine et al., 2002). Quality of life refers to one's personal satisfaction with the life they are living. Being prepared with adaptive coping skills can also help ICD patients minimize the impact of device-specific concerns and enhance their quality of life.

Our minds and our bodies are programmed to respond to a variety of physical, mental, and social stressors. Because stress can manifest in these different ways, it is vital to be prepared with adaptive strategies to respond to those stressors. If we are not armed with effective coping strategies, it is easy to see oneself as a victim of our experiences. It is not uncommon for ICD patients to feel victimized by their heart problems and treatment experiences. Some may even view their device as an unwelcome reminder of their condition. This pattern of thinking can lead to the development of anxiety. Anxiety is a basic emotion that we all experience from time to time. While anxiety is an emotion that is both natural and necessary for healthy functioning, it is important to recognize when anxiety becomes maladaptive, or in other words, when it begins to have a negative impact on your daily lives. Anxiety can be experienced in three different types of symptoms; cognitive symptoms like your thoughts or fears, behavioral symptoms such as your actions or responses, or physical symptoms such as bodily sensations.

Patients living with an ICD often experience a variety of anxiety symptoms. About 13 to 38% of patients experience significant symptoms of anxiety (Sears et al., 1999). The most common anxiety symptoms for ICD patients include thinking negatively or fearfully about the device, avoidance behaviors, and bodily hypervigilance. Fear is certainly an understandable experience for the ICD patient, given the potential for something as unique as ICD shock. As humans we tend to fear the unknown; the unpredictability of the shock experience and the aversive nature of pain can certainly lead someone to fear the potential for shock. However, most patients report that shock is not significantly or lastingly painful. So while a patient might have a natural tendency to think the experience of shock might be very negative, the reality is that it is typically described as just being startling or surprising.

Many patients attempt to act in certain ways that they think will reduce their chances of receiving a shock. This often includes avoidance of particular situations, objects, or activities. While these avoidance behaviors reflect an attempt for control of a seemingly uncontrollable situation, this often leads to deficits in quality of life and even more distress and fear. This is particularly true for patients who avoid perceived triggers that were previously very positive experiences – such as the child who avoids sleepovers for fear of having a shock at someone else's home, or the young adult who chooses to leave college after having been shocked on campus, or the husband who avoids hugging his wife or children for fear of hurting them in the event of a shock. It is important to realize that avoidance is an entirely ineffective strategy! An ICD can fire at any time, in any place, in any situation, making the avoidance of perceived triggers a hopeless effort.

Bodily hypervigilance simply refers to paying excessive attention to one's bodily symptoms. Patients with ICDs who exhibit hypervigilance may constantly scan their bodies for any changes in physical sensations that they believe may signal an impending shock. However, much like avoidance, while hypervigilance may help patients feel like they have more control over their device functioning, it is actually a useless strategy for preventing shock.

Depression may be present in about 24 to 33% of ICD patients (Sears et al., 1999). Symptoms of depression can be related to feeling like the device is limiting your ability to function or live life the way you want to. Feelings of sadness, hopelessness, or not enjoying things you once did are also common symptoms of depression. Patients most at risk for developing depression may include those with a history of ICD shock, as they struggle with interpreting their device and treatment experience as something positive.

Proposed Strategies for Success

When you are faced with unique challenges it may be easy to find yourself feeling isolated as you struggle to make sense of your situation. But it is essential to realize that YOU ARE NOT ALONE! Many people coping with ICD treatment experience frustration that they are just not living life the way they want to. Being prepared with effective ways to deal with the stress of ICD treatment is essential in taking control of living life the way you want to. The following strategies emphasize promoting better quality of life while coping with the stress of treatment with an ICD.

1. Develop a shock plan

Because you have an ICD, you are automatically protected from dangerous heart rhythms. Your ICD protects you by constantly monitoring your heart; when the device detects an abnormal rhythm, it delivers a shock that restores normal heart rhythm. Although shock may be something a patient wishes to avoid, shock is an indication that the ICD is doing its job, keeping you protected. It can be helpful to plan ahead for shock, so that you and your loved ones have a clear understanding of how to handle the situation. Having a plan in place ahead of time can reduce some of the stress that may occur after receiving a shock. Discuss developing a shock plan with your healthcare team so that you can feel prepared should you ever experience a shock in the future.

2. Promote family adjustment

Adjustment to life with an ICD takes time. Living with a device may create changes for you or for members of your family. It is normal to feel stress or guilt because of these changes. But it is essential to remember that all families are faced with events that initiate change. Whatever the initiating factor may be, it is important to remember that families are connected as a team. Changes within the family need not be negative. In fact, many patients describe their family as being stronger after dealing with the challenges of treatment with an ICD. Family adjustment is certainly an ongoing process that requires time and energy by all members. It is normal to experience changes in the family, both positively and negatively. Any problems you had before your device implantation are unlikely to have gone away. Being able to talk openly about your feelings can help you to work out solutions together. It is important for all members of the family to identify their needs and acknowledge them by maintaining healthy interests and activities.

3. Take time to relax

Relaxation is the act of letting go of the stress and worry you may be experiencing. Learning effective ways to relax and let go of tension can lead to a sense of calm and serenity. Learning to control your breathing is a powerful tool for relaxation. By focusing your attention on taking slow, deep breaths you can take control of allowing your mind and body to relax. Deep breathing is a tool you can utilize in a variety of settings - during doctor's appointments, lying in bed at night, or in any of the daily situations you find stressful. Identify how you feel after breathing deeply. Make a list of situations in your daily life where breathing deeply may be helpful.

4. Communicate with your healthcare team

Developing effective communication with your healthcare team is a vital component of taking control of your health and well-being. Misunderstandings about the purpose and function of the device are not uncommon. Do not hesitate to ask questions about your ICD, heart condition, or medications. Write questions down ahead of time and bring to your appointments to facilitate communication. Request educational materials from your providers. Being an informed patient will reduce misconceptions about the ICD and may decrease your risk of developing emotional distress. Being proactive about gaining knowledge about your health will help you feel more confident and in greater control of your treatment experiences.

5. Schedule pleasurable events

Part of taking control of your emotional well-being involves intentionally scheduling rewarding activities that you commit to follow through with. It makes sense that when you start doing fun or pleasurable activities you may begin noticing that life feels a little more rewarding again. Identify some activities that you can schedule for yourself to help the good things in your life feel enjoyable again. Make sure you follow through with participating in these activities despite any fear or discomfort.

6. Maintain physical activity

Regular physical activity can improve your health and quality of life in a number of ways. Exercise helps maintain a better mood, assists in regulating biological rhythms, and is a vital component of controlling weight. Routine exercise is also a healthy way to keep stress at a minimum and increase energy. Discuss some physical activities that are safe and enjoyable with your healthcare team. Identify some of the personal benefits you might gain in participating in physical activities.

7. Decide what is really important to you

People who are faced with implantation of an ICD may be forced to look at life a little differently. Studies suggest that individuals with health issues who are able to adjust appropriately actually report feeling more resilient than before their illness. This is the idea of gaining strength through hardship. If a person can navigate the stress of coping with treatment with an ICD successfully by continuing to embrace what is really important to them, the quality of their life can be better than ever. Deciding what is truly important to you – family, spirituality, or anything you find intrinsically rewarding – is a vital step in improving your quality of life.

8. Consult a professional

Even if you know strategies to deal with your difficulties, at times stress can still become too overwhelming to handle on your own. Despite all of your efforts, there are times when stress cannot be handled by one person any longer. When that occurs, seeking the help of a professional is the best way to gain support in dealing with what you are experiencing. It is not uncommon for people dealing with health issues to develop psychological symptoms. Many seek help from a mental health professional in order to better manage or cope with their feelings. It is important to be able to recognize when it may be beneficial to enlist the help of a professional.

Keep in mind that implementing change in your life is a process – it is something that takes time and commitment. Using the skills and strategies outlined in this chapter should provide you with the building blocks to facilitate the process of enhancing adjustment to treatment with an ICD and making changes in your life that you desire. I encourage you to go back and read the material frequently and share what you have learned with your family and friends. I hope that this knowledge, in combination with regular follow-up care by your healthcare team, will help you take control of creating the life that you want to live. Remember that challenges are expected. Coping effectively with treatment with an ICD helps you to change your mindset from being a victim of heart disease to celebrating life as an ICD survivor. I commend you in your ongoing journey and hope that this information helps you take a step forward in facilitating the process of adjustment and creating the quality of life that you desire.

References:

Irvine J., Dorian P., Baker B., O'Brien B.J., Roberts R., Gent M., Newman D., Connolly S.J. (2002). Quality of life in the Canadian Implantable Defibrillator Study (CIDS). American Heart Journal, 144, 282–289.

Schron E.B., Exner D.V., Yao Q., Jenkins L.S., Steinberg J.S., Cook J.R., Kutalek S.P., Friedman P.L., Bubien R.S., Page R.L., Powell J. (2002). Quality of life in the Antiarrhythmics Versus Implantable Defibrillators Trial: impact of therapy and influence of adverse symptoms and defibrillator shocks. Circulation, 105, 589 –594.

Sears S.F. & Conti J.B. (2002). Current views on the quality of life and psychological functioning of implantable cardioverter defibrillator patients. Heart. 2002;87:488–493.

Sears S. F., Todaro J. F., Saia T. L., Sotile W. M., & Conti J. B. (1999). Examining the psychosocial impact of implantable cardioverter defibrillators: A literature review. Clinical Cardiology, 22, 481-489.

Additional Resources:

How to Respond to an Implantable Cardioverter Defibrillator Shock; Samuel F. Sears Jr, PhD, Julie B. Shea, MS, RNCS, and Jamie B. Conti, MD
Available at: http://circ.ahajournals.org/content/111/23/e380

How to Respond to an Implantable Cardioverter Defibrillator Recall; Kari B. Kirian, MA, Samuel F. Sears, PhD, and Julie B. Shea, MS, RNCS, FHRS
Available at: http://circ.ahajournals.org/content/119/5/e189

Coping with my Partner's ICD and Cardiac Disease; A. Garrett Hazelton, MA, Samuel F. Sears, PhD, Kari Kirian, MA, Melissa Matchett, PsyD, and Julie Shea, MS, RNCS, FHRS
Available at: http://circ.ahajournals.org/content/120/10/e73

Sexual Health for Patients with an Implantable Cardioverter Defibrillator; Lauren D. Vazquez, PhD, Samuel F. Sears, PhD, Julie B. Shea, MS, RNCS, FHRS, and Paul M. Vazquez, DO
Available at: http://circ.ahajournals.org/content/122/13/e465

Practical advice from a patient who has been through recovery of a pacemaker and ICD implantation

In no particular order:

- Before surgery, move some of your dishes and glasses at home to shelves where you won't have to stretch to reach. You can use your right arm, but it is less painful to not stretch at all the first few days.

- If you are a woman, consider packing a strapless bra for the hospital. When I got home from the hospital the first time, I put one on and it was so much less painful without the weight of my breasts tugging on the incision. And I am not large or saggy at all. I even slept in mine and it was much more comfortable. For my second surgery, I took one to the hospital and put it on as soon as I was in my room after the procedure.

- Get some of the squooshy pillows...the kind filled with teeny beads that are covered in stretchy nylon. Lots of kids have them and they sell them in fun shapes and colors. They are very lightweight and perfect for molding however you need it. I used one tucked under my slinged arm at night so my elbow was not tugging down the incision site toward the mattress. In fact, I still use one at night when I sleep on my left side as it is just more comfortable.

- If you are not used to sleeping on your back, consider putting a pillow under your knees. I did not feel comfortable sleeping on either side for a while and my back killed me the first night but once I put a pillow under my knees, the pain disappeared.

- Consider having your partner sleep in a different bed for the first two nights. My husband is a flailing sleeper and I was terrified he would whack my incision...he slept in the guest bedroom for a few nights.

- Get a good haircut that does not require you to raise your arm above your head to style. You will still want to look good while recovering. Using the sprayer in my kitchen sink to wash my hair before I was able to shower made me feel so much better.

- Identify clothes from your wardrobe that are easy to put on. My casual summer skirts with elastic waistbands and some shirts that snap on the front were perfect when I had my surgery in the summer. Sweats and a zip-up hoodie were great in the winter. And slip on shoes. Make sure whatever you take to come home from the hospital in fits the criteria. And invest in a front-closure bra for when you eventually put a strapped bra on, it's easier than reaching around back.

- Get out and walk as soon as you feel you can…I even walked around the hospital and it felt good just to move around, even if slowly at first.

- A friend brought by a tray of cut up fruit and veggies after my surgery. It was the perfect food to have around. No prep necessary, no cutting, no anything, just grab and eat…and it was healthy. You might consider fixing up a tray the night before you leave so you will have it when you get home. I recovered at home by myself and formerly easy things, like opening a jar of salsa, were nearly impossible when favoring your left arm.

- My bed is kind of high and I am kind of short. Without the use of both arms to get myself in and situated, I realized it was not that easy. My husband brought me the stepstool from his closet and put it by the bed…perfect for using as leverage to shift my behind farther into the bed once I got in, then I swing my legs up.

- Talk to other people who have been through it…you aren't alone!

Resources

ACHA
(Adult Congenital Heart Association)
6757 Greene Street, Suite 335
Philadelphia, PA 19119-3508
(888) 921-ACHA
http://www.achaheart.org

American Heart Association
7272 Greenville Ave
Dallas, TX 75231
Customer Service
1-800-AHA-USA-1
http://www.heart.org

Brugada Syndrome
http://www.brugada.org

Heart Rhythm Society
1400 K St. NW, Suite 500
Washington DC 20005
(202) 464-3400
http://www.hrsonline.org

Hypertrophic Cardiomyopathy Association
328 Green Pond Rd.
PO Box 306
Hibernia NJ 07842
Phone: 973-983-7429
http://www.4hcm.org

National Institutes of Health (NIH)
9000 Rockville Pike
Bethesda, Maryland 20892
http://www.nih.gov

SADS Foundation
(Sudden Arrhythmia Death Syndromes)
http://www.sads.org

SCAA
(Sudden Cardiac Arrest Association)
1250 Connecticut Ave NW, Suite 800
Washington, DC 20036
Toll-Free: (866) 972-SCAA
http://www.suddencardiacarrest.org

University of Michigan Hospital and Health Systems
Cardiovascular Center
1500 E. Medical Center Dr.
Ann Arbor, MI 48109
888-287-1082
http://www.uofmhealth.org/heart

Congenital Heart Center
University of Michigan Health System
C.S. Mott Children's Hospital
1540 E. Hospital Dr.
Ann Arbor, MI 48109
1-877-308-9111
http://med.umich.edu/Mott/congenital/index.html

Facebook:
(under groups)
Young ICD Connection

Would you like to share your story?

Are you interested in helping others who are new to ICD implantation by sharing your story? Reading about ICD recipients' or supporting family members' experiences can help others who are trying to cope with their own adjustment to living life with an ICD. Maybe you would like to share what you have learned on your journey that would encourage and help others to cope.

We are looking for ICD recipients of any age and/or their family members to submit their personal story for future publications of the *"ICD Connection: A Collection of Patient & Family Stories"*. If so, please contact by e-mail:

Helen McFarland, RN
University of Michigan Hospital
Device Clinic Nurse
hmcfarla@umich.edu

HELEN MCFARLAND

Pictures from Young ICD Connection Conference

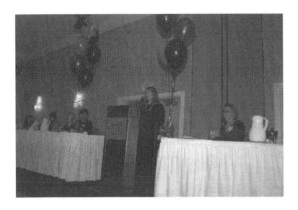

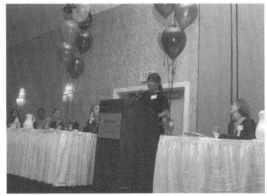

The program begins with young ICD recipients who share their stories*

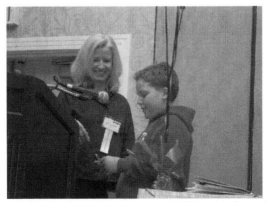

Sarah LeRoy, NP looks on as a young ICD recipient shares his story to the group*

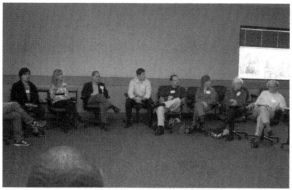

Dr. Gerald Serwer, U of M Congenital Heart Center, joins the "Parents of Children with ICD's" discussion group*

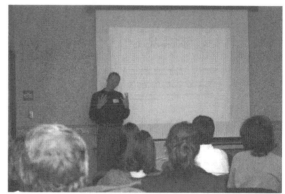

Dr. David Bradley, U of M Congenital Heart Center, lectures on Genetic Testing for ICD patients and families*

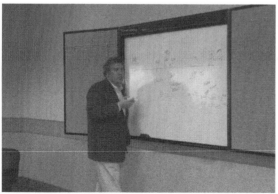

Dr. Frank Pelosi, U of M Cardiovascular Center, lectures on ICD indications*

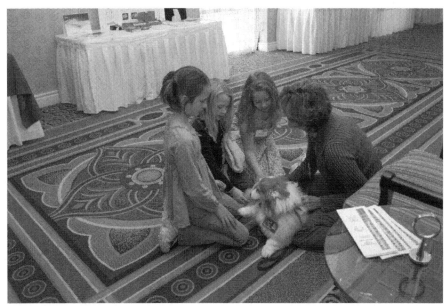

Volunteers from *Therapaws* were available throughout the day*

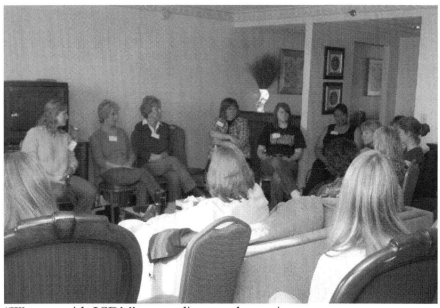

"Women with ICD's" group discuss relevant issues

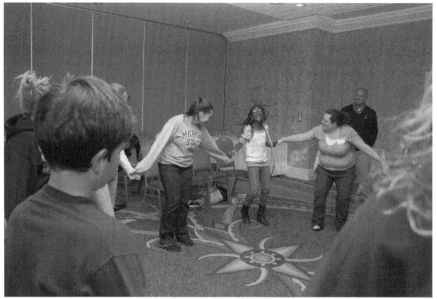

Children and teens enjoy teambuilding games

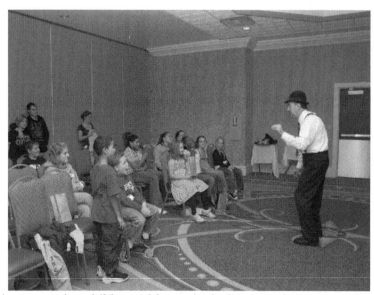

A magician entertains children with magic during a session

Photos reproduced with permission from EP Lab Digest, January, 2009, Vol 9, No 1

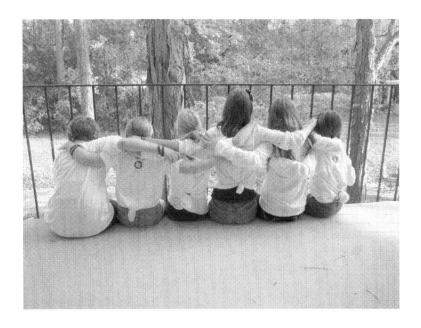

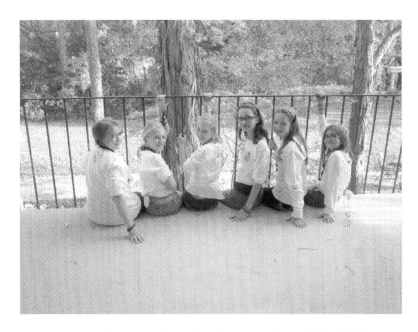

"Enjoying new friends and connecting with old friends!"

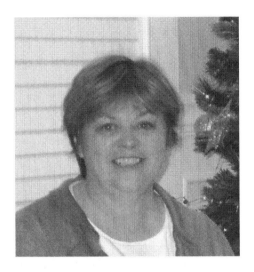

ABOUT THE EDITOR

Helen McFarland has been employed as a registered nurse at the University of Michigan Hospital and Health Systems for over 20 years mainly in the specialty areas of Cardiology and Electrophysiology. Helen received certification from the Heart Rhythm Society as a specialist in cardiac device programming in 2007. In 2011, she graduated from Eastern Michigan University with a degree in Communications. Currently, she is pursuing a Master's Degree in Educational Media and Technology. Helen is the proud parent of an amazing daughter, Ashley Marie. In her spare time, she enjoys traveling and exploring creative arts.

Thank you for taking our survey.

UM Frankel Cardiovascular Center Patient Education Program, enolan@med.umich.edu *or 734-232-4137.*

Please help us improve by telling us what you think. *Your opinion matters to us and to other patients and families.* Please check all that apply and write in your comments in the space provided.

I am:

[ ] ICD patient   [ ] Family of ICD   [ ] HC Provider   [ ] Other
                patient   (faculty/staff)   (describe)

- ❑   Yes, I have read the book.
- ❑   Yes, I have shared the stories with others.
- ❑   Yes, I still have the book.
- ❑   I have a better understanding of life with an ICD.
- ❑   The stories prepare patients/families to live with an ICD.

What I liked best:

What I liked least:

ICD stories/perspectives for future ICD books:

OPTIONAL
Your Name:
Your Phone Number:

If you prefer, you can do this survey online. Go to
http://www.surveymonkey.com/s/K32SQZM

Tear out this page. Fold here, tape, add postage, and mail to address below.

University of Michigan
Samuel and Jean Frankel
Cardiovascular Center
Patient Education Program
Room 2332, SPC 5852 – CVC
1500 E. Medical Center Drive
Ann Arbor, MI 48109-5852

Patient Education Program
UM Frankel Cardiovascular Center
(Attention: E. Nolan)
CVC Room 2332, SPC 5852
1500 E. Medical Center Drive
Ann Arbor, MI 48109-5852